Psychoanalysis, Poetic Testimony, and the Trauma of the Holocau

In this fascinating and innovative book, Rina Dudai looks at Holocaust trauma through the lens of poetic testimony: the act of writing poetry and prose to both relay and process traumatic events.

Dudai begins with a study of both factual testimony and the act of bearing witness in the aftermath of trauma. She uses these as the foundations for her exploration of poetic testimony and the benefits the creator will find over and above other forms of testimony. Showing how this method avoids the additional trauma often brought about by making survivors directly address their experience, Dudai offers a new toolkit to psychoanalysts and psychotherapists working with patients experiencing trauma. Through an analysis of the works of three writers who survived the Holocaust – Primo Levi, Ka-Tzetnik, and Aharon Appelfeld – Dudai establishes a conceptual framework for discussing this mode of testimony and the poetic language through which it speaks. By comparing the work of these writers, Dudai identifies the distinct qualities of this form of poetic language while establishing a foundation for discourse of other literary works that deal with trauma.

Through close textual analysis and the incorporation of therapeutic concepts like "acting out" and "working through," *Psychoanalysis, Poetic Testimony, and the Trauma of the Holocaust* is an invaluable resource to psychoanalysts and other mental health professionals working with trauma patients, as well as students and scholars of literature and 20th-century history.

Rina Dudai is an interdisciplinary scholar of literature, film, and psychoanalysis, based in Israel. She is a member of the interdisciplinary group at the Tel Aviv Institute for Contemporary Psychoanalysis.

Art, Creativity, and Psychoanalysis Book Series

Series Editor: George Hagman, LSCW

The *Art, Creativity, and Psychoanalysis* book series seeks to highlight original, cutting edge studies of the relationship between psychoanalysis and the world of art and the psychology of artists, with subject matter including the psychobiography of artists, the creative process, the psychology of aesthetic experience, as well as the aesthetic, creative and artistic aspects of psychoanalysis and psychoanalytic psychotherapy. *Art, Creativity, and Psychoanalysis* promotes a vision of psychoanalysis as a creative art, the clinical effectiveness of which can be enhanced when we better understand and utilize artistic and creative processes at its core.

The series welcomes proposals from psychoanalytic therapists from all professional groups and theoretical models, as well as artists, art historians and art critics informed by a psychoanalytic perspective.

Affect in Artistic Creativity
Painting to Feel
Jussi Saarinen

Scansion in Psychoanalysis and Art
The Cut in Creation
Vanessa Sinclair

The Story of Original Loss
Existential Trauma in the Arts and Psychoanalysis
Malcolm Owen Slavin

The Psychoanalysis of Aesthetic Experience
Self, Relationship and Culture
George Hagman

For a full list of all titles in the series, please visit the Routledge website at: https://www.routledge.com/Art-Creativity-and-Psychoanalysis-Book-Series/book-series/ACAPBS.

Psychoanalysis, Poetic Testimony, and the Trauma of the Holocaust

Rina Dudai

Routledge
Taylor & Francis Group
LONDON AND NEW YORK

Designed cover image: Moshe Gershuni, *Untitled*, 1989, 120 × 80.

First published 2026
by Routledge
4 Park Square, Milton Park, Abingdon, Oxon OX14 4RN

and by Routledge
605 Third Avenue, New York, NY 10158

Routledge is an imprint of the Taylor & Francis Group, an informa business

British Library Cataloguing-in-Publication Data
A catalogue record for this book is available from the British Library

Library of Congress Cataloging-in-Publication Data
Names: Dudai, Rina author
Title: Psychoanalysis, poetic testimony and the trauma of the Holocaust / Rina Dudai.
Description: New York: Routledge, 2026. | Series: Art, creativity, and psychoanalysis | Includes bibliographical references and index. |
Identifiers: LCCN 2025043074 (print) | LCCN 2025043075 (ebook) |
ISBN 9781032517452 paperback | ISBN 9781032517469 hardback |
ISBN 9781003403753 ebook
Subjects: LCSH: Holocaust, Jewish (1939-1945)—Personal narratives—History and criticism | Holocaust, Jewish (1939–1945), in literature | Psychic trauma in literature | Holocaust, Jewish (1939–1945)—Psychological aspects
Classification: LCC PJ5012.H65 D87 2026 (print) |
LCC PJ5012.H65 (ebook)
LC record available at https://lccn.loc.gov/2025043074
LC ebook record available at https://lccn.loc.gov/2025043075

ISBN: 978-1-032-51746-9 (hbk)
ISBN: 978-1-032-51745-2 (pbk)
ISBN: 978-1-003-40375-3 (ebk)

DOI: 10.4324/9781003403753

Typeset in Times New Roman
by codeMantra

This book is dedicated to my grandmother, Tzila Honigwachs, and my uncles, Emanuel (milosh) and Leo Honigwachs, who were murdered in the Holocaust. And to my uncle, Michael (Mikle) Honey who survived the Holocaust and carried Auschwitz in his heart until his last day.

May their memory be blessed.

Contents

Acknowledgments

I am grateful to Galit Atlas, Neomi Bronfman-Huler, Jose Bruner, Zahava Caspi, Rachel Dagan, Nitza Drori-Peremen, Orit Dudai, Yadin Dudai, Amos Goldberg, Rachel Heiblum, Shlomit Rimon-Keinan, Dan Miron, Pnina Shirav, Yigal Schwartz, and Chana Ulman, who read parts of the manuscript and offered wise and helpful comments.

I am thankful to the Appelfeld, Pagis, and Fink families for generously allowing me to quote from the writings of Aharon Appelfeld, Ida Fink, and Dan Pagis; and to the Gershuni family, particularly Juan Jose Garcia, for the kind permission to feature Gershuni's painting on the cover.

This book is an edited translation of my Hebrew book, *Tongue of Fire: A Poetic Testimony to Holocaust Trauma*, published in 2021 by MOFET Publishing House, Tel Aviv. I wish to express my gratitude to Mofet Publishing House for granting permission for the translation; to Mirjam Hadar and Tali Frastai for translating the text; and to Gissi Sarig for translating Pagis's poems.

My heartfelt thanks go to Routledge, and in particular to Zoe Meyer and Deepika Batra, for their invaluable help and guidance throughout this journey.

To my beloved grandsons, Itay and Ori: I hope that, despite the difficult reality in our beloved homeland, you will find your own paths and meet the high waves of an uncertain future with courage, wisdom, empathy, and hope.

Permissions Acknowledgments

Every effort has been made to contact the copyright holders for their permission to reprint selections of this book. The publishers would be grateful to hear from any copyright holder who is not here acknowledged and we will undertake to rectify any errors or omissions in future editions of this book.

Selected parts from Chapter 1 were published in the following paper and reprinted with the permission of the *Journal of Literature and Trauma Studies*, University of Nebraska Press:

> Rina Dudai, "'And in the Beginning, There Was Oblivion': The Role of Forgetting in Working through the Holocaust Trauma in Poetic Language", *Journal of Literature and Trauma Studies 3:2*, Fall 2014, University of Nebraska Press (2019), 49–72.

Selected parts from Chapter 3 were first published in the following paper and reprinted by permission of *Yod: Revue des etudes hebraiques and juives*:

Rina Dudai, "From Excess to Origin: Traversing Time Zones as an Act of Redemption in the *'The Man Who Never Stopped Sleeping'* by Aharon Appelfeld," *Yod: Revue des etudes hebraiques and juives 19* (2014), 249–258.

Literary Quotations

Excerpts from Dan Pagis, *Poems*, trans. Gissi Sarig (Hakibbutz HaMeuchad, 1991), 206 [Hebrew], in Chapter 1 are reprinted by the kind permission of the Pagis family and ACUM Publishing. All rights reserved.

Excerpts from Ida Fink's short story *Traces* were reprinted with the kind permission of the Fink family and Northwestern University Press. Ida Fink, *A Scrap of Time*, trans. Madeline Levine and Francine Prose (Northwestern University Press [1983] 1995). All rights reserved.

Excerpts from Dante Alighieri, *Inferno*, trans. Robert M. Durling (Oxford University Press, [1321] 1996). All rights reserved.

Excerpts from Paul Celan, *Selected Poems and Prose of Paul Celan*, trans. John Felstiner (Norton, [1955] 2001). All rights reserved.

Excerpts from Aharon Appelfeld *The Searing Light, The Story of my Life, and Essays in the First Person*, translated from Hebrew for this book by Mirjam Hadar, were used with kind permission of the Appelfeld family. *The Man Who Never Stopped Sleeping* © 2009 Wylie Agency (UK) Ltd, also © 2017 Penguin Random House LLC, Schocken House, an imprint of the Knopf Doubleday Publishing Group, a division of Penguin Random House LLC.

Excerpts throughout the book taken from Ka-Tzetnik, *The House of Dolls*, trans. Moshe M. Kohn (Simon and Schuster, [1953] 1955).

Excerpts throughout the book taken from Primo Levi, *If This is a Man, The Truce*, trans. Stuart Woolf (Sphere/Penguin Random House LLC, [1958] 1988).

My thanks go to Faber and Faber for permission to quote lines from Primo Levi Collected Poems (c) 1992.

My thanks go to New York Press for permission to quote from interviews with Primo Levi in the volume edited by Belpoliti and Gordon; to Norton/Liveright (Kindle); and Einaudi Publishing for their permission to quote from Primo Levi's story *Quaestio de Centauris*, trans. McPhee Jenny.

Introduction

On the twentieth anniversary of my father's death – after my brother Giora and I swept his tombstone clean as we do each year, ever loyal to our *Yekke* roots, laid the customary wreath in its place, and lingered around the gravesite together with close friends and family, trying to keep his memory alive – my uncle Michael, my father's brother, and I decided to meet later that evening, once the family gatherings were over, and talk about Michael's life during the years of the war. Motche, as my father was called by everyone, had been the leader of the "Young Maccabee" regiment in Nový Jičín, a city in the Czech Republic (at that time still Czechoslovakia), immigrated to *Eretz Yisrael*/Palestine in 1938 at the young age of 16 through the "*Youth Aliyah*" organization. When he took leave of his family on the platform of the Bratislava train station, he had no idea he would never again see his brothers Imanuel (Milosh) and Leo or his mother Tzila, although the clouds of war were already gathering on the horizon. Excited, he looked forward to a pioneering future of building a homeland for the Jews, of settling the land, and of joining the kibbutz Kfar Ruppin, where my brother and I were later born. After the memorial at the cemetery concluded, several of us met at my mother's house, and although we had planned to talk about my father's achievements and commemorate his endeavors, his pioneering stories remained untold, stowed away in the letters he had written to Halef, one of his six brothers who had himself succeeded in extracting a group of pioneering youth from Czechoslovakia after the invasion of the Nazis and smuggling them to Sudetenland, from where they forged convoluted paths of escape and finally arrived at Palestine – waiting for the moment when someone would agree to take the time to listen to them. Later that evening we met, my uncle Michael and I, in my house in Rehovot. Michael stretched himself out across the couch and began chatting about the usual tidbits of everyday life, and time flew by until, yet again, despite our decision to fully dedicate our evening to a testimony of his memories of the war, we found ourselves approaching midnight with this difficult journey still before us.

We began. "In Auschwitz, all Ten Commandments were broken," Michael said, looking at me with a piercing gaze. His soft, subtle demeanor metamorphosed suddenly, shockingly, into an entirely different one: an emotional figure, contorted by

DOI: 10.4324/9781003403753-1

rage and trapped inside himself; one that I was unable to reach or help. I recoiled. "Michael," I said gently, "maybe we'll set another meeting? It's late, at this hour the carriages turn into pumpkins," feebly attempting some light humor as a way of extricating us from the unfolding situation. Michael, whose face was drained, pale, insisted. At that instant, everything came to the surface – the buried traumas, the unspoken horrors of the past, the gaping sense of loss – searching desperately for a way out. But I shrank away and into the sofa, and despite having long awaited the moment when we could dedicate our time and full attention to this testimony, I deferred. Michael, who at the start of the evening had looked young for his age, full of joy and calm, was exhausted; the bypass surgery he had recently undergone was visible on his face. Standing at the threshold, terrified of the powerful forces that might erupt, uncontrolled, I ended the meeting and promised another one in the near future. As I accompanied him to his car and wished him well on his way home, throwing in the family's mandatory "drive carefully," I said goodbye – albeit with a heavy heart and concern for his mental and physical state, which had transformed him so suddenly. Was it the right thing to do, I wondered, to open things up again? Michael, one of the survivors among the hundred children who served as Josef Mengele's "runners" in Auschwitz, had already given testimony in 1995 as part of the Spielberg project in London, where he was living at the time. His wife, also a survivor, adamantly refused to discuss her past and did not allow him to give his testimony at home, requiring him to walk to the house of friends in order to tell his story before the camera. After her death, Michael immigrated to Israel, where he lived from 2006 until his death in 2010.

I spent a sleepless night deliberating whether to press on with the journey into Michael's personal testimony. First, I worried about Michael's physical and emotional state. What if, despite the fact that he had carried the heavy burden of massive, ongoing trauma on his shoulders for so many years, his heart would no longer be able to withstand it, and something inside him would break? I felt I wasn't qualified to undertake the task alone. It seemed irresponsible and wrong. But then again – was it solely concern for Michael that had led me to avoid listening to his testimony? Or was I hiding behind a high-minded explanation, while in fact I myself was incapable of crossing the threshold of the witness into a realm that demands focused, attentive listening to such incomprehensible evil?! "I will need to clarify this point," I told myself, and fell into a restless sleep, from which I was interrupted by a desperate knocking at my door. I glanced at the clock on the bedside table. It was 6:10 am. I jumped out of bed and ran to the door, as horrific scenarios rushed through my head: something terrible has happened to Michael! The worst has happened; Michael is dead! A voice yelled from the other side of the door: Call an ambulance! Someone's lying on the side of the road… Here, in this quiet suburban neighborhood, at the foot of a hill with just a single road passing through, I panicked. "Michael," I whispered to myself. Michael, just not this. The thought that he might have been lying there all night, and I hadn't known about it, drove me crazy. Barely managing to find my phone, I dialed emergency services, submitted a confused report about an incident, and ran outside. On my way to the group of people huddled around, I scanned the road and saw no sign of Michael's car. Gradually, I came to realize that this was not about Michael; that he did, in fact, manage to get home safely. Several days later, I discovered that a man whom I had not known had died of cardiac arrest during his morning run just outside my house. It took me many more days to calm down. Looking at that day from a distance, however, I couldn't ignore two themes that would turn into the core of this book. Michael, whose heart stopped forever in 2010, never did give his testimony to me, despite both of us wanting to do so, despite the fact that here in Israel he had borne witness in lengthy historical detail on camera for *AMCHA*.[1] It seems that Michael was destined to spend his life circling around the core of his trauma, telling and not telling it, trapped forever in its jaws. And I, who so yearned to be a witness to his personal story, the story that hadn't been told, could not endure to hear it: at the moment of truth, I deferred the testimony to a later time, one that never came to pass.

For years I've been studying poetic ways of coping with Holocaust trauma. I wrote my PhD thesis on the poetic modes used by Aharon Appelfeld, Ka-Tsetnik, and Primo Levi, whose paths of struggle I tell in this book. Nevertheless, something in the unmediated encounter, devoid of all poetic defense mechanisms, between the survivor bearing witness, Michael, and the receiver, me, was so threatening, so unbearable, that this unique personal testimony has remained mute. The story buried at the core of the trauma refused to reveal itself.

In this book, I examine the language of poetic testimony – that which does expose itself, the language that has traversed "the thousand darknesses of death-bringing speech," in the words of Paul Celan, that "went through it and could emerge, 'enriched' by it all,"[2] which came out with no words to describe what had taken place but was nevertheless written, subtly and quietly, in order to constitute a new meaningful reality. What is the nature of this poetic tongue of testimony? What is its power in relation to other testimonial tongues? Do different artists choose different poetic strategies? These are the questions I try to answer in this book.

Notes

1 AMCHA is a non-profit organization that provides services to Holocaust survivors and their families. I would like to thank the late Yoram Amit from AMCHA Rehovot, who dedicated many hours to empathetic and caring listening to Michael's testimony.

2 Paul Celan, *Selected Poems and Prose of Paul Celan*, trans. John Felstiner (Norton, 2011), 395.

Part One

The Primal Scream and the Silence

Chapter 1

Absence as the Language of Trauma[1]

On June 7, 1961, in Session No. 68 of Adolf Eichmann's trial held in Jerusalem, the Polish-born writer and Holocaust survivor Yehiel Dinur – also known by his pen name, Ka-Tzetnik 135633 (or simply Ka-Tzetnik)[2] – was called to the witness stand to give testimony about his experience in Auschwitz:

> I was there for about two years. Time there was different from time here, on Earth. Every fraction of a second rotates there on a different gear. And the residents of this planet did not have names; they had neither parents, nor children [...] they [...] breathed according to other laws of nature [...] their names were the Ka-Tzetnik numbers [...] I see them, they are watching me, I see them, I saw them next to the line [...].[3]

As it became apparent that the witness was drifting into incoherence, the presiding judge intervened, attempting to redirect him to focus on factual testimony, but Dinur stumbled off the witness stand and fainted. The sitting was adjourned, and Dinur was taken to the hospital.

Among the many testimonies given during Eichmann's trial, this episode seared itself most deeply into the collective Israeli consciousness. Ostensibly, it is odd that this moment – in which Dinur ended up *not* telling his story – would come to represent the traumatic experience of millions of Holocaust victims. However, it is precisely from its collapse into silence that Dinur's testimony derives its power: the presentation of the witness's inability to put the event into words conveyed the horror of the experience more authentically than any detailed factual account could ever have.[4] This moment of breakdown brings to the fore the muteness that lies at the heart of the survivor's trauma, as acknowledged by the Italian survivor-writer Primo Levi: "[...] those who saw the Gorgon have not returned to tell about it, or have returned mute."[5]

The silence at the core of traumatic experience has been conceptualized by various scholars over the past decades. Jean-Louis Lyotard defines this silence as a *differend*: that linguistic state in which that which should be expressible becomes impossible to articulate.[6] Lyotard uses Auschwitz as a reference point for traumatic experiences that give rise to such an inability to establish coherent and cohesive

DOI: 10.4324/9781003403753-3

expression. For him the silence that surrounds the phrase "Auschwitz was an extermination camp," as he writes in *The Differend*, is not a state of mind; it is the sign that something remains to be phrased, which is not.[7] Lyotard claims that in such traumatic experiences, the traditional categories of conceptualization are insufficient, and any attempt to assign preconceived distinctions to the event robs it of its singular essence. Giorgio Agamben also acknowledges the inadequacy of language to represent the Holocaust, calling attention to the *lacuna* that lies at the core of Holocaust testimony. In *Remnants of Auschwitz*, he notes that survivors bear memories so traumatic that they cannot express them even to themselves. Therefore, he suggests that listening to a survivor's testimony requires a unique kind of attention, one that focuses on the *lacuna* itself and takes this absence into account.[8] Dominick LaCapra builds on these concepts and others in developing his concept of *excess* to describe the unarticulated remnant that lies at the heart of a traumatic experience, defying attempts at representation in language or other symbolic systems.[9] Time and again, the story of the surviving witness is described as haunted by the inability to find words to express it.

Nevertheless, the compelling human imperative to express, communicate, and transcribe the horrific events has led many survivors to attempt to put their experiences into words. Writing, however, is difficult for those who experienced the trauma of the Holocaust. Transcribing testimony requires a reengagement with death, a willing return to and immersion in unimaginable realms of human evil. This forces the survivor-writer into finding ways to contend with unresolvable struggles between powerful opposing forces, among them the struggle between writing and living, the struggle between authenticity and representation, and the struggle between the primal scream and the silence.

In his book *Literature or Life*, Jorge Semprun succinctly describes these struggles as a choice between writing and living, a choice in which he chooses amnesia in order to heal and survive. This intended election of life over writing turns out, however, to be temporary. Later on in the book, Semprun lays out the paradox he repeatedly confronts but never manages to resolve: He had nothing but the experience of his own death to tell the story of his life and to go on living it through writing. But writing dragged him back into death, trapping him in it.[10]

Once the decision to put testimony into writing is taken, the writer finds himself confronted with additional difficulties: by putting the concrete, sensual experience of horror into words, the survivor-writer finds that some of the authentic immediacy and essence of the experience is inevitably lost. This loss is twofold. On the one hand, the futility of any attempt to convey the concrete, sensual experience of horror through language is exposed in all its hopelessness. Indeed, how can one possibly express, in words, the all-pervading odor of the camps? Semprun writes that these doomed efforts conveyed his most personal memory, distinguishing him everywhere from others, a memory that was burning within him with a flame of horror and baseness, leaving a smell of burned flesh. He felt a day would soon come when there would be no one left to carry the actual memory of that smell. Only poetry would remain, he argued, a literary reference, the idea of a smell.[11]

At the same time, Semprun expresses despair that the reader would never truly comprehend his experience. Everyone knows what smoke is, or at least thinks they know, but they will never know; they cannot imagine it no matter how sincerely they want to.[12]

Calling forth the horror of trauma by literary and poetic means is the foremost challenge that lies before the survivor-writer. *Only the primal scream emerging from deep within the gut*, he writes, *only the silent voice of death, could possibly express the suffering.*[13]

The primal scream and the silence: the challenge of representing in language the unrepresentable trauma, the *lacuna*, and the *excess* that evades representation is at the heart of this book. While the attempts of Holocaust survivors to tell their stories are varied, they share this common struggle to represent the mute core of trauma through text. The mechanisms they find in poetic language for coping with these intense conflicts, for keeping the tensions alive while restraining their destructive power, lead them to create a unique language: a poetic language of absence.[14]

Absence as Buried Memory

The existence of the traumatic core as absence, concealing itself from its own subject, is vividly described in the poem "17" written by Israeli poet Dan Pagis:[15]

17

Brain, pleased, surveys his centers:
A center for speech, a center for lies,
A center for memory
(seventy clocks, at least, each keeping its own time),
A special center for pain –
Suddenly
(Who is speaking, please? Who's there?)
He is stunned by the astonishing news:
There is a hidden circle
Whose center is everywhere
And whose circumference is nowhere;
A center which is so close
That he will never
Be able to see it.[16]

In this poem, the brain surveys its various functional centers. In the course of the survey, the brain moves from the "speech" center to the "lies" center – namely, the center of poetic language – and then moves on to the centers of "memory" and "pain." Beyond these centers, however, an "astonishing," paradoxical bit of news is revealed: "There is a hidden circle/Whose center is everywhere / And whose circumference is nowhere; / A center which is so close / That he will never / Be able to see it." Beyond the important centers enumerated by the brain, which all participate in constructing one's self-identity, a hitherto unknown entity is revealed: a circular, all-encompassing and yet utterly invisible one. Although it remains nameless, this is the center of absence, a demarcated periphery which leaves traces but evades all signifiers. It is the *lacuna*, the *differend*, the *excess*: a void that allows nothing to penetrate, existing unto itself, complete but indescribable.

Tracing the trajectory of the brain's survey of itself, we discover yet another phenomenon. Some of the centers are familiar ones, which the brain recognizes with "satisfaction," fully aware of their existence and enjoying their activity. The speech center, the lies center, and the memory center fall under this category: domains that deal with representation. And indeed, speech, fiction, and memory are all languages in which the brain is fluent. The fourth line, "seventy clocks, at least, each keeping its own time," echoes the fact that these are different languages.[17] After the linguistic clarifications, the brain moves on to examine the pain center, and finds it belongs to an entirely different category. All at once, a sense of the measurable passage of time vanishes, and the speaker, surprised by someone speaking, asks the mysterious voice to identify itself. In lieu of an answer, the paradoxical hidden circle is revealed. The trajectory from the centers of the various languages, through pain, to the hidden circle – the domain of absence – is significant. Pain has a different ontological status: it is not a center of *representation* but rather of *presentation.* As such, it stands apart from the other centers of language. Unlike the various languages, pain is not abstract but physical and sensory. Perhaps it is already located in the domain of the unconscious, where things happen suddenly, without awareness or foresight: "Suddenly / (Who is speaking, please? Who's there?) / He is stunned by the astonishing news." Even the poem's use of punctuation points toward a separate, parenthetical level of existence. Only from this alternate plane of pain can the speaker proceed into the all-encompassing domain of absence.

Pagis describes this hidden circle as one that exists simultaneously alongside the brain's other centers. Unlike the other centers, he does not explicitly identify or name this just-discovered center. It is, rather, circumscribed through a chain of paradoxes: it is "everywhere" but "nowhere"; so close that it is invisible. The circle is an all-encompassing totality but simultaneously inconceivable and impenetrable. Its most prominent feature is its existence as an unknown, an absence. This image is a vivid depiction of the preliminary state of trauma: a state in which the traumatic event is preserved, untouched and unknown, in the realm of oblivion as a nuclear core into which nothing can penetrate, but whose presence is nevertheless felt in all other domains by means of traces that testify to its buried presence.

A Struggle with the Memory of Trauma: Oblivion, Forgetting, Confronting

The language of absence upholds a dialogue with the memory of trauma in a variety of ways. I will elucidate these approaches through an analysis of several poetic texts. The poems "Small Poetica" and "The Tale," both written by Pagis, demonstrate the poet's dialogue with oblivion; "Traces" by Ida Fink shows the struggle between memorializing and forgetting; and finally, Pagis's text "Gravity" depicts his confrontation with the trauma.

Oblivion

Small Poetica

You're allowed to write everything,
like that, and that,
You're allowed with all the letters you find,
With all the signs you plant among them.

It's worth checking, of course,
If the voice is your voice
And the hands are your hands.

If so, imprison your voice,
Gather your hands, and heed
The voice
Of the empty page.[18]

Sidra DeKoven-Ezrahi claims that Pagis's poetics dissolves the boundary that separates the living from the dead and presence from absence, a boundary that the survivor-writer attempts to traverse.[19] And indeed, the *ars poetica* poem "Small Poetica" illustrates the process of the unraveling of language from words, through sounds and punctuation marks, and finally to the raw material of the blank page itself. The writer embarks on his poetic journey from a preliminary state in which a broad reservoir of linguistic possibilities is open to him: "You're allowed to write everything," including free-standing sounds[20] and even punctuation marks: "all the signs you plant among them." As the poem unfolds, the range of possibilities shrinks and the act of writing is reduced. The original license to write "everything" is revealed to be deceitful, and is replaced with a demand for authenticity. This demanding entity orders the writer to imprison his voice, to gather the hands that write, and to heed the mute voice of the *empty page*. The trajectory of the evolution from writing, through the gathering of the hands that write and the imprisonment of the voice, to a deference to the silence of the blank page itself, is especially intriguing. Writing, a means for representing reality, is converted into a physical voice, which is in turn replaced by the absent voice of the empty page: in following this transformation, we witness the unraveling of representation.

The writer is commanded to leave the page blank at the end of this process after his own authenticity is questioned: "It's worth checking, of course, / If the voice is your voice / And the hands are your hands." Why does a fidelity to authenticity require the page to remain empty? Here we find that the poem vividly plays out the confrontation between the impulse for representing the traumatic experience through language with an opposing desire, which aims not at the representation of the traumatic experience in language, but rather at the presentation of the absence itself, a physical expression of the muteness of the raw material: the empty page. Speech, as a form of verbal representation, is liable to damage the authenticity of the experience and must therefore be rejected; only the void of the blank page is able to truly codify the core of the traumatic memory in the most well-preserved and protected place, its own body.

"Small Poetica" brings to the fore the urgent need for authenticity by ordering the writer to heed the voice of the empty page, as the only possible true expression of the traumatic core. Another poem by Pagis, "The Tale," returns to the motive of the empty page and takes it a step further, representing in language the act of lingering over the page:

The Tale

Once I read
A tale about a grasshopper just a day old,
A green adventurer, who at dusk
Was devoured by a bat.

Immediately afterwards, the wise old owl
Gave a short condolence speech and said:
A bat would like to make a living too,
And there are many other grasshoppers in the meadow.

Immediately afterwards came
A last empty page.

Forty years since that moment
I am hunched over that page,
I do not have the strength
To close the book.[21]

The poem attempts to call forth the traumatic core, while simultaneously monitoring and restraining it, by employing two distinct poetic devices. The first device makes use of the parable genre, which sets the traumatic memory in a conceptual, schematic world, where it is uprooted and detached from any context. The creation of this artificial distance thus allows the subject to observe and relay the traumatic event while disconnecting from the authentic experience. The second part of the poem abandons the generic narrative of the fable genre and instead offers an alternative route: a text that delves into an authentic and immediate experience, adhering to the sensory experience of the body drowning in the empty page, thereby evoking a genuine sense of the traces of the trauma while preventing its content from surfacing into conscious memory.

The distinction between these two strategies is emphasized by the poem's structure, which is separated into two clear sections. In the first section, the writer recites a parable he once read mechanically, almost childishly; in the second section, he is found to be frozen in place, bent over an empty page at the end of the book that he is unable to close. The first section has the qualities typical of a fable: a short, didactic story aimed at conveying a concise moral principle. The power of the parable resides not in its description of characters but in the universal and timeless knowledge it bequeaths, and therefore the particular details of the tale are insignificant. The parable related in the poem tells the tragic tale of a young and innocent grasshopper, barely out in the world, who by nightfall is devoured by a bat. The second verse is dedicated to a wise owl who gives a short consolation speech that touches upon the travesty of the grasshopper's death but nonetheless evokes mitigating arguments for the insect's demise: "A bat would like to make a living too / And there are many other grasshoppers in the meadow." The parable ends with a sense of closure and a moral advocating an acceptance of the world order, for all its apparent injustices.

The poem's second section abruptly abandons the parable genre, traverses the mythical time of the story, and homes in on the physical, concrete medium of the book itself: "Immediately afterwards came / A last empty page." The transition from the familiar, archetypical content of the parable to the physical dimensions of the book containing it, and finally to the blank last page that literally closes the book spurs a process of deconstruction that shatters the familiar and reliable framework set up at the beginning of the poem. The writer's prolonged lingering over the book's final empty page opens a window onto another dimension of experience and makes present the pain and loss of personal trauma. This open-ended lingering is offered by the poem as an alternate, subversive moral to the parable, in the form of a stubborn refusal to come to terms with the horror of murder and the act of aggression. The defiance is not presented as heroic or stemming from a dramatic source of strength but as human: "I do not have the strength / To close the book."

As such, the poem's final stanza transforms the refusal to close the book into a manifestation of "acting-out" that resurrects the traumatic past in an ongoing present, reinvigorating the memory by persistently remaining hunched over the blank page and refusing to move on. Acting-out is an impulsive action taken by the subject, in which he is trapped in the circle of trauma.[22] The fixation on obsessive repetition blocks the possibility for properly processing the experience and obstructs the construction of a distance that would allow for an analytic observation of and control over the trauma.[23]

In the text of the poem, the narrator indeed testifies directly to his inability to process the trauma. "Processing" is a therapeutic concept in which the past is reconstructed in a controlled and supervised way and is thus not experienced anew in its full intensity.[24] In the work of processing, the subject reaches emotional insights, a sort of rational understanding of emotions that is possible only when the subject is at a safe distance from the traumatic memory. From this vantage point, it is possible "to understand, to see, to articulate, and to control that which was previously unacknowledged, unseen, unspoken, and unacted."[25] The narrator's inability to close the book testifies to the fixation that prevents him from processing the traumatic memory: his urge to linger within the recurring experience of the authentic memory, shrouded in oblivion, renders him incapable of moving on.

"The Tale" was written in 1985, and it demarcates a period of forty years in which the narrator has been hunched over the blank page. Taking this into account, the forty years referred to in the poem are those between 1945, the end of the war, and 1985, but they also call attention to another alternate time – the vicious circle of trauma. Closing the book would signify a coming to terms, a reconciliation which the narrator is unable to accept.

One could say that on the poetic level, Pagis found a fascinating way to contain the uncontainable, to make-present the acting-out, and in his quiet and subtle way, even to put forth an alternative mode of coping. He dismantles the parable's conventional story-scheme: he begins with an archetypical schematic parable pattern, one with which he has been familiar since childhood. As the poem progresses, the parable metamorphoses into a universalized narrative – into *the* tale. It contains the injustice found in the parable's conventional mold and thus reinforces the unbearable truth. The alternative tale, the one undermining the process of coming to terms with injustice that is offered in the poem's first section, is the tale of this particular narrator, the one who carries infinite pain, whose strength is diminishing, so much so that he is unable to close the book. The narrator's unique story rips apart the universal one, shattering and undermining it. By acting-out and making present the inability to process traumatic memory, the poem exposes the absence, the *lacuna*. On the level of psychological processing, it offers no closure, no salvation; instead, it posits a refusal to be consoled. At the same time, poetic language makes use of this act of defiance to outline, in language, the unrepresentable boundaries of the traumatic core.

Poetic language works at the liminal peripheries of language.[26] From this precarious position, it challenges the concealing mechanisms of memory and language, takes them apart, and pries open a crack through which the traumatic world can be glimpsed. At the same time, poetic language goes beyond allowing a glimpse into the core of the trauma; it also has the generative power to reconstruct the shattered world and give it new expression.

Forgetting

Recent research on memory has claimed that the most authentic memories are precisely those that have not been remembered or activated.[27] Evidence shows that the more often a memory has been evoked, the further it deviates from the authentic original experience. With every activation, the memory is liable to be tinted by the colors of the context in which it is evoked and to undergo alterations in light of the conditions of its activation. Thus, it is in fact the memory that has been long buried and forgotten, that has not been activated or used at all, that is the closest to original impressions of the constitutive experience, and that is most vibrant and alive. Conversely, the work of processing memories inherently entails the creation of a certain distance from the original experience. Even the processing of grief, for example, can under certain conditions be experienced as a betrayal of the lost object, since the process is inextricably bound up with assimilation and effacement.[28]

With these findings in mind, I approach the non-story of the trauma. Paradoxically, it is the non-story – the mute, concealed, unremembered story – which is the most authentic one. However, a story that is not told remains inaccessible; authentic, perhaps, but doomed to languish in oblivion. The literature of testimony thus upholds the tension between the preservation of the authenticity of the non-story by keeping it silent and the obsessive need to bring the story to light, to retrieve it from oblivion and tell it in the most accurate detail possible, in order to keep the memory alive. A vivid example of the tension between the non-story and the obsessive need to tell it can be found in the short story "Traces" by Ida Fink.[29]

The story begins with a woman who is presented with a photograph that evokes in her the memory of a traumatic event in which she witnessed children and their parents shot to death by the Nazis:

> Yes, of course she recognizes it. Why shouldn't she? That was their last ghetto. The photograph, a copy of a clumsy amateur snapshot, is blurred. There's a lot of white in it; that's snow. The picture was taken in February. The snow is high, piled up in deep drifts. In the foreground are traces of footprints; along the edges, two rows of wooden stalls. That is all. Yes. This is where they lived. She recognizes those stalls; they used to be market stalls and were converted to living quarters. Well, perhaps she has put it badly, they were simply enclosures made with boards.[30]

The photograph is apparently not in good shape. Damages of first, second, and third orders make identification difficult: the low quality of the photograph taken by an amateur photographer on the one hand and its traumatic content on the other. Moreover, the photograph is in fact not an original, but a copy. The conditions of the event itself add on to these difficulties. The photo shows white snow piled high along the road, on which it's possible to discern only traces of human footprints. The language of absence in the story is encompassed in this single snapshot. The snow holds the outline of the footprints of those who are no longer. "The people are gone – their footprints remain," says the woman.[31] The absence, unseen and unheard, can only be perceived through the footprints, the traces left behind. A trace, in this sense, is both ontological, a sign left behind by the absent, and a mark circumscribing, making present, the absence itself. Without the outline provided by the footprints, there would be no way of knowing of the existence of the absence.

In her seminal book *On Photography*, Susan Sontag writes that photography "is like a footprint or a death mask."[32] Sontag conceives of the photograph via two paradigms that, she claims, characterize the intimate relationship between the photograph and reality: footprints and the death mask. These two paradigms express, above all other images, the paradoxical proximity of the photograph to the language of absence. According to Sontag, by virtue of being the most direct connection to the original object, the photograph represents it in the most concrete fashion. Nevertheless, despite its concreteness, the photograph is also, at the same time, the closest living testimony to the absence of the original object. This contradictory relationship is brought even more closely together by Roland Barthes. In his book *Camera Lucida*, Barth describes the photograph as adhering tightly to its origin, fully united with and inseparable from the original: "[…] they are glued together, limb by limb […]."[33]

The photograph in the story "Traces" serves not just as a trigger for accessing the traumatic memory. It also provides a site for the reconstruction, the making-present, of the forgotten event. The act of identifying the photograph's content metamorphoses into an act of reconstructing the scattered fragments of the traumatic core story. The process of calling forth the memory is gradual, accompanied by an ongoing struggle with the strong impulse to forget. After carefully observing the photograph and noting the precise location of the photographer who took the picture, the speaker pushes it away and says, "I prefer not to be reminded…."[34] Later on, after the speaker indirectly makes clear that the footprints imprinted on the snow are those of people who were shot, and after she begins to tell the details of the event, she says again, "I prefer not to remember."[35] Nevertheless she continues, since she feels that only her testimony can provide the living traces for the traumatic event: "But suddenly she changes her mind and asks that what she is going to say be written down and preserved forever, because she wants a trace to remain."[36] Thus, the concrete visual photograph of footprints in the snow is converted into a verbal expression of the story, which, via the written record, becomes the trace of memory.

Fink embarks on the trauma story by describing the photograph in words. The transference of the trauma's forgotten story into the space of the snapshot allows her to begin to unearth the hidden core of trauma. From this point onwards, the obstacle recedes, and the copy of the blurry photograph taken by a clumsy amateur comes to life and appropriates for itself not just the space but also the entire story concealed within the footprints. The black and white photograph becomes a dynamic movie, in which the victims and the executioners move toward their preordained destinies. The film is even accompanied by a soundtrack: "they heard the rumbling, a horse cart drove up to the yard, and on it were the children"; the executioners, talking to the children; the silence of the victims. Even the subdued emotional reaction of the speaker during the act of remembrance is heard: "The first tears, instantly restrained."[37]

The progress of the story is shaky, spiral rather than linear. The speaker moves hesitantly, one foot after the other, toward unearthing the story, then recedes two steps backward, retreating inwards in order to avoid a confrontation with the trauma. The snapshot, now the arena where the struggle takes place, awakens the traumatic memory, excavates it from its state of oblivion, and drags it into the present. The experience of the trauma is relived in full and vivid force. This daunting process threatens the narrator, and in the end the most horrifying part remains untold: "In a calm voice she asks for a short break. With an indulgent smile she rejects the glass of water they hand her. After the break she will tell how they were all shot."[38] The story at the core of the trauma remains mute and recedes back into the darkness of oblivion. The traumatic story thus turns on itself and is transformed into a different tale: one about a momentary encounter with a memory, in which the barrier of oblivion is temporarily opened, and present time and the time of the trauma merge, but only for an instant, before once again separating as the memory sinks back behind the barrier, leaving behind only its traces. "Traces" is about the inability to tell the story – and perhaps also about the adamant refusal to betray the memory, preferring to leave it authentic and untouched; powerful and destructive, but still alive.

> Gravity / Dan Pagis
> If I go down into the valley, I will disappear. The dead area will swallow me up. I will, therefore, skip over it, I'll jump from cliff to cliff. At the very least, from one treetop to another. I decide this – and at that moment, the devil be damned, my grasshopping powers abandon me, and gravity attacks me, pulling me down into the dead area, to its every tiny, neglected recess.
> I take out a measuring tape, rolled up like a snail, I begin to crawl, measuring the crevices, the gorges, the ravines, the folds of the earth – the scope of the porous world. Here it is, spread before me, a living plane.[39]

In her article about Dan Pagis's writing, DeKoven-Ezrahi notes that toward his death, Pagis began writing segments of prose as told by a remembering entity.[40] "Gravity," written in 1982, is among these. DeKoven-Ezrahi interprets the change in the poet's work toward the end of his life as having great significance, testimony that the "sophisticated evasion" that had so characterized his writing throughout his life finally gave way to an autobiographical directness. In her opinion, this shift in style and genre expressed a deep internal revolution, a sort of religious conversion signified by the transition from writing poetry to prose, as well as by other changes in theme, tone, and visual language.[41]

In the poem "Gravity," the urge to skip over the "dead area" is overruled by another force, that of gravity itself, "pulling me down into the dead area"; a force that draws the speaker precisely into the dark recesses of the underworld that threaten to swallow the subject and annul him, which he has tried so hard to evade. Once there, the speaker proceeds to survey it:

> I take out a measuring tape, rolled up like a snail, I begin to crawl, measuring the crevices, the gorges, the ravines, the folds of the earth – the scope of the porous world. Here it is, spread before me, a living plane.[42]

The speaker's rolled-up measuring tape is compared to a snail hesitantly emerging from his house. At this point, the speaker seems to merge with his own measuring tape, becoming the snail who wanders through the void of the world: "the crevices, the gorges, the ravines, the folds of the earth – the porous world." These geographic sites share common characteristics: their structure includes a *lacuna*, an interior void, which the snail is able to measure. The act of measuring takes place only after the snail has stepped out of his house, which he nevertheless carries with him on his travels. The snail's measurements, making present the absences, revive the area. Measuring the absent spaces of the valley (a reference to the "Vision of the Valley of Dry Bones") helps him to turn the "porous world" into a plane. Paradoxically, life is made possible only by inadvertently falling into the abyss and by the slow, painstaking process of taking its measurements. The happy-go-lucky grasshopper, who once bypassed the abyss by hopping over it, is now a snail crawling slowly and meticulously on its underbelly inside the dead area; and through its slow and steady measuring, the snail is able to convert the abyss into a living plane.

Authentic testimonies, whose echoes and voices are one and the same, are those that incorporate within their own core an essential *lacuna*, rather than try to fill or ignore it. Pagis insists on maintaining this absence and time and again demands its presence and representation. The survivor holds in his heart a testimony – a testimony of the absence.

Notes

1 An earlier version of this chapter can be found in my article: Rina Dudai, "And in the Beginning, There Was Oblivion: The Role of Forgetting in Working Through the Holocaust Trauma in Poetic Language", *Journal of Literature and Trauma Studies* (2019), 49–72.
2 *Ka-Tzetnik* is Yiddish for "Concentration Camp Inmate," deriving from *ka tzet*, which was the abbreviation for Konzentrationslager. 135633 was the *ka tzet* number assigned to Dinur in Auschwitz.
3 Yehiel Dinur, "The Testimony of Yehiel Dinur", in *Attorney General of the Government of Israel vs Adolf Eichmann – Testimonies* (The Public Affairs Department of the Prime Minister's Office, 1963), 1122–1123. [Hebrew].
4 Specifically, its collapse in the arena of the courtroom makes it all the more powerful. See: Rina Dudai, *Modes of Coping with Trauma in Holocaust Literature (A. Appelfeld, Ka-Tzetnik, P. Levi)* (PhD dissertation, Hebrew University, 2000), 92–98; Shoshana Felman, *The Juridical Unconscious* (Harvard University Press, 2002), 135–137.
5 Primo Levi, *The Drowned and the Saved*, trans. Raymond Rosenthal (Summit, 1988), 83–84.
6 Jean-François Lyotard, *The Differend: Phrases in Dispute*, trans. Georges Van Den Abbeele (University of Minnesota Press, 1988), 56–57.
7 Lyotard, *The Differend*, 56–57.
8 Giorgio Agamben, *Remnants of Auschwitz* (Zone Books, 1999).
9 Dominick LaCapra, *Writing History, Writing Trauma* (John Hopkins University Press, 2001).
10 Jorge Semprun, *Literature or Life*, trans. Linda Coverdale (Viking Press, 1997).
11 Semprun, *Literature or Life*.
12 Semprun, *Literature or Life*.
13 Semprun, *Literature or Life*, 182.
14 Dudai, "And in the Beginning."

15 Dan Pagis, a Holocaust survivor, was imprisoned as a child in a concentration camp in Transnistria, where he had experiences that he chose never to share.

16 Dan Pagis, *Brain 17*, in *Poems* (Hakibbutz Hameuchad, 1991), 206. [Hebrew]. Translated by Gissi Sarig; I am grateful to Sarig for translating the poems by Pagis that appear in this book.

17 According to the story of the Tower of Babel as it appears in Genesis, God divided the people into seventy linguistic groups, unable to understand one another, and scattered them throughout the world.

18 Pagis, "Small Poetica", in *Poems*, 228, trans. G. Sarig.

19 Sidra DeKoven Ezrahi, "Dan Pagis – Out of Line: A Poetics of Decomposition", *Prooftexts 10:2* (1990), 335–363.

20 In the original Hebrew, the word "that" is a letter diacritic added onto the beginning of words and pronounced "she" (with a short e sound). This word-sound, which signifies the beginning of the unraveling, is also the sound that represents the onomatopoeic request for silence. The double meaning of this sound – signifying a search for something tangible, and simultaneously calling for silence – vividly embodies the struggle which the poem is about.

21 Pagis, *The Tale*, in *Poems*, trans. G. Sarig.

22 Sigmund Freud, "Remembering, Repeating and Working-Through", in *The Standard Edition of the Complete Psychological Works, Vol. 12: The Case of Schreber, Papers on Technique and Other Works*, ed. and trans. James Strachey (Hogarth Press, [1959] 2001).

23 Matthew Erdelyi, *Psychoanalysis: Freud's Cognitive Psychology* (Freeman, 1985); Freud, "Remembering"; Jean Laplanche and Jean-Bertrand Pontalis, *The Language of Psychoanalysis*, trans. Donald Nicholson Smith (Norton, 1973); Saul Friedländer, "Trauma, Transference, and 'Working Through' in Writing the History of the 'Shoah'", *History and Memory 4:1* (1992), 39–59.

24 Processing is considered to be the added value of the psychoanalytical transformation, a change derived from the deciphering of resistances, a liberation from repetitive and destructive patterns, and insights into the emotional dimension. Freud referred to the work of processing as the process through which the past is reconstructed in memory, rather than perpetually present, relived, or acted out.

25 Hans W. Loewald, "On the Therapeutic Action of Psychoanalysis", *International Journal of Psycho-Analysis 41* (1960), 16–33.

26 Julia Kristeva, *Revolution in Poetic Language*, trans. Margaret Waller (Columbia University Press, 1984).

27 See for example: Yadin Dudai, "The Neurobiology of Consolidations, or: How Stable Is the Engram?", *Annual Reviews of Psychology 55* (2004), 51–86; Daniel L. Shacter, *The Seven Sins of Memory: How the Mind Forgets and Remembers* (Mariner Books, 2002).

28 Jacques Derrida, *Memories for Paul de Man* (Columbia University Press, 1986); also, see LaCapra, *Writing History*, 49–50.

29 Ida Fink was born in Zbaraz, Poland, and was 18 years old when the Germans invaded the country. Fink spent two years in the Zbaraz ghetto before managing to escape with her sister. Eventually the sisters immigrated to Israel, where Fink began to write stories based on her own experiences as well as those related to her by others.

30 Ida Fink, *A Scrap of Time*, trans. Madeline Levine and Francine Prose (Northwestern University Press, [1983] 1995), 135–137.

31 Fink, *Scrap of Time*, 135–136.

32 Susan Sontag, "The Image-World", in *On Photography* (Doubleday, 1990), 154.

33 Roland Barthes, *Camera Lucida: Reflections on Photography*, trans. Richard Howard (Hill and Wang, 1980), 5–6.

34 Fink, *Scrap of Time*, 136.

35 Fink, *Scrap of Time*, 136.
36 Fink, *Scrap of Time*, 136.
37 Fink, *Scrap of Time*, 137.
38 Fink, *Scrap of Time*, 137.
39 Pagis (1991).*Gravity*. In *Poems*, 257. [Hebrew]. Translated by Tali Frastai.
40 Sidra DeKoven-Ezrahi, "You Ask How I Write?", *Alpayim 10* (1994), 94–110. [Hebrew].
41 DeKoven-Ezrahi, "You Ask How I Write?", 101–102.
42 Pagis, "Gravity", in *Poems*, 257.

References

Agamben, Giorgio, *Remnants of Auschwitz* (Zone Books, 1999).

Barthes, Roland, *Camera Lucida: Reflections on Photography*, trans. Richard Howard (Hill and Wang, 1980).

Derrida, Jacques, *Memories for Paul de Man* (Columbia University Press, 1986).

Dinur, Yehiel, "The Testimony of Yehiel Dinur", in National Directorate, ed., *Attorney General of the Government of Israel vs Adolf Eichmann – Testimonies* (The Public Affairs Department of the Prime Minister's Office, 1963), 1122–1123.

Dudai, Rina, *Modes of Coping with Trauma in Holocaust Literature* (A. Appelfeld, Ka-Tzetnik, P. Levi) (PhD dissertation, Hebrew University, 2000).

Dudai, Rina, "And in the Beginning, There Was Oblivion: The Role of Forgetting in Working Through the Holocaust Trauma in Poetic Language", *Journal of Literature and Trauma Studies 3* (2019), 49–72.

Dudai, Yadin, "The Neurobiology of Consolidations, or: How Stable Is the Engram?", *Annual Reviews of Psychology 55* (2004), 51–86.

Erdelyi, Matthew, *Psychoanalysis: Freud's Cognitive Psychology* (Freeman, 1985).

Ezrahi, Sidra DeKoven, "Dan Pagis – Out of Line: A Poetics of Decomposition", *Prooftexts 10:2* (1990), 335–363.

Ezrahi, Sidra DeKoven, "You Ask How I Write?", *Alpayim 10* (1994), 94–110.

Felman, Shoshana, *The Juridical Unconscious* (Harvard University Press, 2002).

Fink, Ida, *A Scrap of Time*, trans. Madeline Levine and Francine Prose (Northwestern University Press, [1983] 1998).

Freud, Sigmund, "Remembering, Repeating and Working-Through", in James Strachey, ed. and trans., *The Standard Edition of the Complete Psychological Works, Vol. 12: The Case of Schreber, Papers on Technique and Other Works* (Hogarth Press, [1959] 2001), 147–156.

Friedländer, Saul, "Trauma, Transference, and 'Working Through' in Writing the History of the 'Shoah'", *History and Memory 4:1* (1992), 39–59.

Julia, Kristeva, *Revolution in Poetic Language*, trans. Margaret Waller (Columbia University Press, 1984).

LaCapra, Dominick, *Writing History, Writing Trauma* (John Hopkins University Press, 2001).

Laplanche, Jean and Pontalis, Jean-Bertrand, *The Language of Psychoanalysis*, trans. Donald Nicholson Smith (Norton, 1973).

Levi, Primo, *The Drowned and the Saved*, trans. Raymond Rosenthal (Summit, 1988).

Loewald, Hans W., "On the Therapeutic Action of Psychoanalysis", *International Journal of Psycho-Analysis 41* (1960), 16–33.

Lyotard, Jean-François, *The Differend: Phrases in Dispute*, trans. Georges Van Den Abbeele (University of Minnesota Press, 1988).

Pagis, Dan, *Brain 17*, in Sarig Gissi ed. and trans., *Poems* (Hakibbutz Hameuchad, 1991), 206.

Pagis, Dan, *Small Poetica*, in Sarig Gissi ed. and trans., *Poems* (Hakibbutz Hameuchad, 1991), 228.

Pagis, Dan, *The Tale*, in Sarig Gissi ed. and trans., *Poems* (Hakibbutz Hameuchad, 1991), 243.

Pagis, Dan, Gravity, in Sarig Gissi ed. and trans., *Poems* (Hakibbutz Hameuchad, 1991), 257.

Semprun, Jorge, *Literature or Life*, trans. Linda Coverdale (Viking Press, 1997).

Shacter, Daniel L., *The Seven Sins of Memory: How the Mind Forgets and Remembers* (Mariner Books, 2002).

Sontag, Susan, "The Image-World", in *On Photography* (Picador. Farrar, Straus and Giroux, 1990), 151–180.

Chapter 2

Poetic Testimony of Holocaust Traumatic Memories

What Is Poetic Testimony?

Over the course of the 20th century, and especially following the Holocaust, the act of bearing witness became a fundamental component in the establishment of collective memory, and survivors of extreme events were often called upon to recount the suffering they underwent and the cruelty they witnessed.[1] Scholars researching the act of bearing witness have distinguished between various forms of testimony, some even including accounts beyond the testimonies given by the survivors themselves. In his book *Remnants of Auschwitz*, Giorgio Agamben discusses several types of witness.[2] He notes that Latin distinguishes between *testis*, which refers to "the person who, in a trial or lawsuit between two rival parties, is in the position of a third party," and *superstes*, which "designates a person who has lived through something, who has experienced an event from beginning to end, and can therefore bear witness to it."[3] Dori Laub goes on to name three distinct levels of witnessing: "being a witness to oneself within the experience; witnessing other people giving testimony; and reflectively witnessing the testimonial process itself."[4]

Scholars from a variety of disciplines in the humanities and the social sciences have attempted to conceptualize testimony through extensive research, establishing a conception of the act of bearing witness that lies beyond the factual-scientific discourse. Prominent philosophers such as Jean-François Lyotard and Agamben, researchers of literature and psychology such as Judy Herman Lewis, Shoshana Felman, and Dori Laub, and historians like Dominick LaCapra all recognize the act of bearing witness as a representation of the unique mode of crisis inherent in expressing intense traumatic experiences such as the Holocaust and highlight the frequent failure of language to express the horror. Agamben's *lacuna*,[5] Lyotard's *differend*,[6] and LaCapra's *excess*[7] – these various terms all refer to the black hole at the heart of the testimony; the language of absence into which language collapses, in which the survivor is at a loss when attempting to represent or express the experience. Lyotard notes this clearly when he claims that the essence of bearing witness is found in scattering traces and signs that serve to make-present that which is inexpressible in language. The psychoanalytical discourse of trauma has

DOI: 10.4324/9781003403753-4

heavily influenced the discourse on Holocaust testimony, leading to a portrayal of the breakdown of testimony as a stage in an ongoing work of processing: when the event actually occurs, it is registered but not claimed in consciousness and is only validated in retrospect, years later, by looking back at and reflecting on (to use Freud's term, *Nachtraeglichkeit*) the horror.[8] This psychoanalytical model emphasizes the clinical and therapeutic dimensions of the act of bearing witness.

Other scholars push back against the psychoanalytical conceptualization of bearing witness, contending that the retrospective therapeutic approach to testimony fails to recognize the active and urgent role bearing witness plays in the present. Historian Amos Goldberg[9] and political theorist Michal Givoni[10] highlight the ethical responsibility of witnesses. Givoni claims that approaching the act of bearing witness from within the framework of trauma discourse defines the testimony as subjective and singular and ignores the fact that the testimony is not just a channel for the expression of that singularity but also a moral and political practice. She transcribes the discussion of the survivor's testimony to the observing witness who preserves it, and by doing so draws a distinction – in contrast to Lyotard – between two types of testimony, which, in her opinion, require different practices of bearing witness. While psychoanalytical testimony aims to help the trauma victim process traumatic events, the humanitarian testimony, she claims, aims toward creating a factual and public documentation of the events themselves, one that is an objective, scientific, and emotionally distant representation.[11]

Between these two practices of bearing witness – the tangible, singular, personal testimony that makes-present its own representational failure and is thus always a "retrospective" validation of the catastrophic event, and the objective, documentary, humanitarian testimony that serves as an ethical and political act in the present – I propose a third path: the poetic testimony. This form of testimony is neither disciplined by psychotherapeutic discourse nor by legal, historical, or academic discourse. Poetic testimony, bridging the gap between the singular and the collective, the personal and the documentary, requires a unique practice of its own.

Poetic testimony works through a dual code that allows it to call forth and express the moments of fracture that cannot be represented. Poetic language, in its unique capacity to bear contradictory twists and turns, manages to contain the shards of a fractured world and to use them to construct spaces in which the excess – that which cannot be represented without shattering the text – is able to exist. Poetic language penetrates the flickering material of the catastrophic experience and finds a way to express that which cannot be represented. Paul Celan, in his acceptance speech for the Bremen Literature Prize, said:

> It, the language, remained, not lost, yes in spite of everything. But it had to pass through its own answerlessness, pass through frightful muting, pass through the thousand darknesses of death-bringing speech. It passed through and gave back no words for that which happened; yet it passed through this happening. Passed through and could come to light again "enriched" by all this. In this language I

> have sought, during those years and the years since then, to write poems: so as to speak, to orient myself, to find out where I was and where I was meant to go, to sketch out reality for myself.[12]

In his unique language, Celan highlights the steps of impoverishment: opposite the horror of reality, words fall one by one into silence. But going through this muteness leads, in the end, to another kind of writing, one which is able to reconstitute a new reality. Through this new reality, constructed in poetry, Celan is able to discern where he is and where he is going.

Poetic language is committed to those things buried in the unconscious, hidden from the eye, that are revealed only when a crack opens wide and the concealed world of chaos is glimpsed. Lyotard conceives of these "things" as a voice with its own acoustics, leading those exposed to it into an alternate realm, the realm of the Real: "About the thing [...] it is true that it commands, but it doesn't ask for anything [...] It does not speak at all."[13]

Testimony that speaks in the poetic language of moments of crisis, especially those of Holocaust experiences, calls forth traumatic memories in a unique manner. It allows us to touch the sweltering core of the traumatic experience and to give it form. The memory of trauma is a type of phantom that is almost impossible to grasp but nevertheless cannot be banished. Poetic testimony allows these ghosts to continue to exist and to manifest the traces of an unregistered memory, lingering as a bothersome and ever-present excess, as a sensation that cannot be pinned down and defined. At the same time, this type of testimony carries out the work of anamnesis, which – in an infinite process – listens for signs and makes-present the traumatic memory that anticipates its representations and activates a sense of moral obligation toward this kind of memory. Poetic testimony works in the margins of language, in its liminal areas, and as such, it is able to contain within itself the paradoxes of life and death. By translating the present-absent experience into poetic devices, poetic testimony of extreme situations becomes in and of itself a carrier of memory, transferring the traumatic experience to future generations and enabling additional audiences to join in the work of processing by attentive listening.[14]

Poetic testimony expresses itself in a fragmentary fashion. The shards, the shattered fragments, and the rhythmic and structural caesuras manifest in a form of expression in which we will always remain with a wordless excess, one that refuses to reveal itself and relentlessly harasses us and causes us discomfort. Celan, in his speech "The Meridian," tries to define this aspect of poetry:

> The poem, unmistakably shows a strong bent toward falling silent [...] the poem holds on at the edge of itself; so as to exist, it ceaselessly calls and hauls itself, from its Now-no-more back into its Ever-yet.[15]

Inspired by Celan, I attempt to weave threads between the experience of trauma and the language of poetry, which is, for me, the epitome of poetic language. The trauma speaks from the "edge of itself" because at the heart of the traumatic experience there is an impenetrable excess that is nevertheless present, which can speak – if at all – only from its own margins, from the subtle and fleeting place of the "Now-no more" to the "Ever-yet." This voice is the excess, the metonymic relic that speaks the world of chaos. These fragile threads require a certain kind of attentiveness, a poetic one that captures the unconscious and speaks it. It anticipates that which lies just beneath consciousness, rumbling and allowing us to feel, to touch, perhaps even to see something from the essence of the traumatic experience. This is an attentiveness that traps the unspoken excess – the absence, lacuna, or differend – within the folds and creases of language.

The gaze of poetic language in general, and of poetic testimony in particular, is not direct. Looking into the chaos is dangerous, and if it is to survive, the gaze must pass through a protective shield of poetic devices, a "language grating" (Paul Celan's *Sprachgitter*). In the Greek myth of Perseus and Medusa, the legendary Greek hero Perseus was commanded to behead the Gorgon Medusa, who turned anyone who looked at her to stone. He succeeded by using a "mirror shield" that Hermes, herald of the gods, gave him before embarking on his mission. By using this ruse, Perseus was able to evade the danger of looking directly at the monster; he killed her by looking at her reflection instead and returned home victorious. Poetic language offers just such a reflective shield: it allows us to look at the Gorgon and continue to exist without turning into stone, without collapsing into the void.

While poetic language comes close to the essence of the real and allows us to gaze, albeit indirectly, into the "death-bringing" core of the trauma, it simultaneously places us at a safe, protective distance and sets up a homeostatic system of checks and balances that allows us to call upon the horror without being swallowed by it. The poetic text as testimony is a space in which the traumatic event is conjured in a dose that can be withstood. It is responsible for creating what Edward Bullough calls an "aesthetic distance," the monitoring mechanism that regulates the distance from the lived experience.[16] This mechanism aims to surface the core of the trauma without being consumed by it. As with ceremonies and rituals – and psychotherapy – the poetic work allows for the surfacing of the most threatening elements while observing them from a safe distance.

The Dual Code of Poetic Testimony

Poetic testimony of traumatic experience contains a dual dimension, as two opposing forces are simultaneously at work. On the one hand, the force that strives for contact with the sweltering core of the fractured experience pulls the text toward the core of the trauma; on the other hand, the force attempting to preserve and protect the collapse into this core pushes away, toward an external perspective of constraint. One force attempts to free itself from the burden of linguistic conventions and to arrive, through the cracks, within a hair's breadth of the chaos, as the threat of the collapse of language hovers above; the opposing force creates an organizing framework that contains the process, controls it, and prevents such a collapse. Thus, the closer we get to the traumatic core and the more the threat of erupting forces increases, the more heavily the text relies on poetic devices to keep watch and ensure the unity and survival of the poetic text.

This proliferation of poetic devices constitutes the mechanism of restraint in the text, its preserving foundation, a bedrock that functions as a kind of gatekeeper, working to regulate the resources of energy and to reestablish an equilibrium of forces, thereby allowing the intense experience to be represented. Thus, the restrained style of a linguistic work representing a traumatic memory is not just a rhetorical, stylistic, or aesthetic device but also a textual representation of the mechanisms that work to manage the anxiety that inevitably arises. In other words, the restrained quality of the poetic text is an expression of the system of balances working within the text itself, a homeostatic system that transforms the traumatic experience into language. An inverted relationship is established between an excess of emotions, which demands representation, and the representation itself. The style of restraint becomes, in this respect, an indicator of the metaphoric "capability" to govern the destructive forces, to contain them, and to impose a new order on the chaotic world that asks to be represented. This type of equilibrium system is responsible for ensuring that the primal scream that asks to be represented in the text is not heard "as madness, or worse, as inauthentic, fake," in the words of Aharon Appelfeld.[17] One might assume that this type of equilibrium system is uncontrollable, but in the poetic domain, it can be employed deliberately, at least in part. True expression of the scream requires it to be enveloped in a protective layer. The text presents us with these contrasting forces – those of destruction and those of preservation – not separately, but as an equilibrium. Thus, the presence of restraint indicates the traces of the trauma while simultaneously allowing the trauma itself to be processed.

Poetic-Textual Defense Mechanisms

Although the concept of restraint is familiar among the characterizations of writing styles, there is no theoretical literary model that places restraint at its foundation.[18] I suggest that in the textual representation of traumatic experience, textual restraint is not just a writing style but is foundational, providing the control mechanism necessary for the expression of the erupting and destructive forces of trauma.

In borrowing the paradigm of "psychological defense mechanisms" from the domain of psychotherapy in order to examine "poetic textual defense mechanisms," an analogy between a person and a text is assumed.[19] Such an analogy between a text and a human being is not new. Socrates compared the rhetorics of a memorized text – a speech of an orator – and a living creature, based on their unity.[20] In *The Poetics*, Aristotle claims that a unified plot, similar to an animal, requires a principle of continuity that includes a beginning, a middle, and an end.[21] In these examples, the analogy between a human being and a text is forged based on the formal structure of a coherent, unified organic entity. In the modern period, psychoanalysis contributed an additional dimension for correlation between a person and a text: the dynamic structure of therapy can be compared to the plot structure of a story.[22] The affinity between text and the psychoanalytical process was significantly reinforced by Jacques Lacan, who claims that the text as a whole speaks in the language of the unconscious.[23]

Building on this analogy, I take a closer look at the language of the unconscious, seeking the parallels between psychological defense mechanisms and what I term "poetic-textual defense mechanisms." Psychology offers the concept of defense mechanisms as one part of a system of checks and balances through which personal identity is construed. Freud offers several models of monitoring mechanisms that supervise the transition of unconscious forces to consciousness. Jean Laplanche and Jean-Bertrand Pontalis define the Freudian model of defense mechanisms as a "group of operations aimed at the reduction and elimination of any change liable to threaten the integrity and stability of the bio-psychological individual."[24]

The fundamental idea behind the various forms of this psychoanalytic model is the existence of two opposing psychological forces: the repressive and the repressed. The form taken on by their struggle and the relative success of each force determine the mental health of an individual. According to Freud, defense mechanisms prevent aggressive libidinal drives from surfacing into consciousness and allow the ego to navigate between the demands made by the id and the Superego as well as those made by reality. Thus, they serve a homeostatic function of maintaining an equilibrium in the individual's mental economy of drives and emotions and protect the individual from impulses that might lead to a collapse of the self.[25]

In the following chapters, I will show how the style of restraint works in text in a way similar to that of psychological defense mechanisms in that it spreads a security net that protects the unity and stability of the text. The function served by the style of restraint in a highly charged narrative text is not just aesthetic, as one might assume, but also plays a crucial role in the text's own survival, preventing it from shattering. Assuming that a text's style of restraint participates in its own maintenance of control, one could also assume, to a certain extent, a metaphoric correlation to a person's defense mechanism, which aids in the confrontation of a phenomenon, despite its intensity. My assumption is that whatever monitors the text can be referred to as "poetic-textual defense mechanisms," minimizing the influence of components that threaten the unity and stability of the text while allowing for the expression of the unspoken excess that demands to speak the traumatic experience. Poetic expression of this mechanism can be found in Nathan Alterman's poem "The Foreign Poem," when he addresses the power of the poem:

> It is stronger than me! Its *defenses*, fading in despair,
> will rise up before me.[26]

The arsenal of psychoanalytic discourse offers two central patterns of defense: "acting-out" and "working through."[27] Acting-out is an impulsive act of the subject that makes-present the traumatic past within the present by reviving it through action. The subject does not remember the experience in his consciousness, in his declarative memory; rather, he revives and enacts the conflictual situation in which it is bound. In fact, he remembers nothing of that which was repressed and forgotten but acts in light of the implied, hidden memory of the experience.[28] When the subject is trapped in the circle of trauma, he is unaware of the origin of the action and its meaning. The materials of acting-out are obsessive, mechanical, and melancholic repetition of the past. This repetition bars the way to adequate processing of the experience and prevents the creation of a distance from which the traumatic experience can be analytically observed in a controlled fashion.[29] Acting-out can be considered a defense mechanism in which the unconscious protects itself from being revealed by the ego, part of the mechanisms of repression and denial. Freud conceives of acting-out as an action that distinguishes between the conscious and the unconscious, whose goal is to signal something, to leave traces of something that strives to express itself. In his article "Remembering, Repeating and Working-Through," Freud writes:

> the patient does not remember anything of what he has forgotten and repressed, but acts it out. He reproduces it not as a memory but as an action; he repeats it, without, of course, knowing that he is repeating it.[30]

Working-through, in contrast, is a means of processing past memories through consciousness. According to Freud, working-through aims to defy the tendencies of denial, repression, and compulsive repetition held by traumatic memories by means of the creation of adequate distance from the memory that allows a comprehensive understanding of the past. This, in turn, allows the patient to overcome resistance to change, resulting in proper functioning in the present.[31] Working through trauma involves reconstructing the past in a controlled way, ensuring that the past is not experienced anew in its full intensity. This work creates the conditions for more appropriate use of the defense mechanisms and for the observation of the past from a critical perspective, a place of sublimation, which allows a revitalization of life in the present.[32] Processing includes a conscious acknowledgment of the mechanisms of denial, which aids the subject in freeing himself from the mechanical grasp of the past. In working through trauma, the subject creates a sort of rational understanding of the emotion,[33] made possible by the existence of an "aesthetic distance"[34] from the traumatic memory. This is a distance from which one can understand, see, speak, and control what was hitherto unseen, undefined, and unspoken.[35] Processing is considered to be the added value of the psychoanalytic transformation, derived from the de-codification of resistances: a liberation from familiar patterns of compulsive repetition.

La Capra goes a step further and distinguishes between the primary memory of trauma and the secondary memory of one.[36] A primary memory, according to La Capra, belongs to the person who lived through the events and remembers them in a certain way. This memory is authentic and forceful, but it includes errors, which arise from the denials and repressions typical of these memories, among other reasons. A secondary memory is the result of critical work on the primary memory, work that is carried out by the person who experienced it or by an observer or witness of second order, such as a historian or an artist. The person who underwent the experience and the observer meet on the plane of the secondary memory, where they can agree on a shared representation of the experience that solidifies the precise memory. If the trauma is re-experienced as part of acting-out, a process of working-through is required in order to transfer the primary memory into a memory of second order.[37] According to La Capra, the historian's mission should not be full, empathic documentation, which would revive the other's traumatic memory in its full force, but rather a restrained, subdued recording of the memory. The process requires a more subtle delivery of the traumatic nature of the event, rather than a full-blown recreation of it.[38]

In this book, I extend the range of usage of the concepts "acting-out" and "working-through" beyond the domains of history and psychotherapy and into the domain of literary textual analysis. These concepts, borrowed from the realm of psychotherapy, allow me to characterize poetic texts that cope with the traumatic memory of the Holocaust and examine various manifestations of the style of restraint as a textual defense mechanism.

Poetic defense mechanisms can be found in the physical shields of Ancient Greek literature, such as the one in the myth of Perseus and Medusa mentioned previously. A variation of this theme appears in the Iliad, in the story of the Shield of Achilles.[39] After Achilles is stripped of his armor, his mother turns to the artist Hephaestus to forge a shield for him that would protect him when he returns to battle. The artist creates a shield that includes a reflection of every detail of the world, in essence bearing witness to the world in all its horrific elements of war and cruelty, while simultaneously defying this world by protecting its owner.[40] This same dynamic can be found in the literary text: it dares to reflect the horror while allowing one to observe it from a protected space, that aesthetic distance that prevents the observer from collapsing into the horror.[41]

In the following chapters, I will examine these poetic defense mechanisms according to four organizing principles of poetic devices that participate in the construction of an impression of restraint in the text: the principle of amount (expansion or contraction); the principle of distinction (sharpness or blurriness); the principle of cohesion (convergence or division); and the principle of value assignment (hierarchy or equivalation).[42] These principles are responsible for overseeing the text and for regulating the emotional intensity inherent in the essence of bearing witness to a catastrophic experience. The representation of traumatic memory in poetic testimony requires, I claim, a dual-acting mechanism: on the one hand, one that directs its gaze toward the heart of the trauma, and on the other, one that creates a linguistic grating through which it is possible to observe the trauma without collapsing into it. This dual mechanism allows the construction of reality through language, a construct that imposes order on the observed chaos.

Spectator of a Shipwreck:[43] The Testimony of the Addressee

This book began with an MA thesis[44] that dealt with Aharon Appelfeld's magnificent book, *Searing Light*. During the time spent writing my thesis (1980–1982), when the subject of trauma had not yet come to the fore of literary-cultural research, I felt there must be a deep connection between the intense experiences of the author and the work's subdued forms of structural and stylistic representation. What struck me most in recurring readings of Appelfeld's work was the contrast between his stylistic restraint and the intensity of the experiences described in the texts. I tried to make sense of this contrast by carefully examining linguistic-poetic appearances in the text. The thesis concluded that the restraint was not just a stylistic phenomenon but also an expression of the Herculean struggle taking place within the writer's spirit, a struggle between forces striving to break out and express the extreme experience on the one hand and counter-forces attempting to subdue and control them. In my doctoral thesis, I went on to address this question by drawing on discourses from other disciplines: psychoanalytic discourse and that of the aesthetics of the sublime, two fields which came together in the 1990s to form a prominent field in the disciplines of humanities, social sciences, and cultural studies: trauma studies.

This book addresses the matter of trauma representation in poetic language. An analysis of the poetic devices employed in the representation of trauma allows me to follow the ways in which poetic testimony constructs a site where psychological defense mechanisms of writers and readers alike encounter what I refer to as poetic-textual defense mechanisms and how these latter have the power to enable poetic testimony of the writer as well as the reader, the addressee. These mechanisms are broadly explored in the following chapters by means of textual analyses of three writers: Aharon Appelfeld and his books *Searing Light* and *The Man Who Never Stopped Sleeping*[45]; Ka-Tzetnik and his book *The House of Dolls*[46]; and Primo Levi and his book, *If This Is a Man*.[47] This continuum expresses a range of textual modes for processing the traumatic events experienced by all three writers: from an expression dictated by the memory of the body (Appelfeld), through the exploding expression of the primal scream (Ka-Tzetnik), to an expression dictated by the rational foundations of the witness, observing from an aesthetic distance (Levi). Each analysis will examine the writer's unique style and offer an interpretation of their poetic-textual defense mechanisms.

I undertake this analysis from the vantage point of a "spectator of a shipwreck," to use the poignant metaphor coined by Hans Blumberg,[48] as a distant observer of a catastrophe playing out in the horizon. By examining the poetic testimony of those who were able to confront the trauma of the Holocaust and to represent it in their work, I offer a mode of bearing witness to traumatic events that is able to present, preserve, and transmit the horror of trauma without collapsing into itself and to bridge the gap between the singular, psychological need for processing and the collective, historical need for documentation: poetic testimony.

Notes

1 Avishai Margalit, *The Ethics of Memory* (Harvard University Press, 2002).
2 Giorgio Agamben, *Remnants of Auschwitz: The Witness and the Archive* (Zone Books, 1999), 17.

3 Agamben, *Remnants*, 17.
4 Shoshana Felman and Dori Laub, *Testimony: Crises of Witnessing in Literature, Psychoanalysis and History* (Routledge, 1992), 75–76. See also: Chana Ullman, "Bearing Witness – Across the Barriers in Society and in the Clinic", *Psychoanalytic Dialogues 16:2* (2006), 181–198; Dana Amir, *Bearing Witness to the Witness: A Psychoanalytic Perspective on Four Modes of Traumatic Testimony* (Routledge, 2018).
5 Agamben, *Remnants*.
6 Jean-François Lyotard, *The Differend: Phrases in Dispute*, trans. Georges Van Den Abbeele (University of Minnesota Press, 1988).
7 Dominick LaCapra, *Writing History, Writing Trauma* (John Hopkins University Press, 2001).
8 For more on this matter, see for example: Cathy Caruth, ed., *Trauma: Explorations in Memory* (Johns Hopkins University Press, 1995); Cathy Caruth, *Unclaimed Experience* (Johns Hopkins University Press, 1996); Amos Goldberg, *Trauma in First Person: Diary Writing during the Holocaust* (Indiana University Press, 2017).
9 Goldberg, *Trauma in First Person.*
10 Michal Givoni, *The Ethics of Witnessing: A History of a Problem* (Hakibbutz Hameuchad, 2015). [Hebrew].
11 Givoni, *Ethics of Witnessing.*
12 Paul Celan, "Speech on the Occasion of Receiving the Literature Prize of the Free Hanseatic City of Bremen", in *Selected Poems and Prose of Paul Celan*, trans. John Felstiner (W. W. Norton, [1958] 2001), 395–396.
13 Jean-Francois Lyotard and John Ronan, *Anamnesis of the Visible* 2 (University of Nebraska Press, 1999), 27. https://www.jstor.org/stable/20686094.
14 For more on this, see Rina Dudai, "Trauma in Translation: Crossing the Boundaries between Psychoanalysis and Film", *Projections 8:1* (2014), 41–60.
15 Paul Celan, "The Meridian, Speech on the Occasion of Receiving the Literature Prize of the Free Hanseatic City of Bremen", in *Selected Poems and Prose of Paul Celan*, trans. John Felstiner (W. W. Norton, [1958] 2001), 409.
16 Edward Bullough, "Psychical Distance as a Factor in Art and an Aesthetic Principle", *British Journal of Psychology 5:2* (1912), 87–118.
17 Aharon Appelfeld, "Beyond Tragedy", in *First Person Essays* (World Zionist Organization, 1979), 49. [Hebrew].
18 A comprehensive discussion of pathos and anti-pathos can be found in: Rina Dudai, "Study of Poetic Devices that Convey Restraint in the Charged Narrative Text" (MA Thesis, Tel Aviv, 1983), 7–18. [Hebrew].
19 The term "text," as I employ it in this book, is an inclusive term that incorporates a triad of interactive components, which together grant the text its "life." These include the text itself, the author who writes it, and the reader who responds to it.
20 Plato, *Phaedrus*, eds. Alexander Nehamas and Paul Woodruff (Hackett, 1995), section 264C. Socrates claims that "every discourse must be organized, like a living being, with a body of its own, as it were, so as not to be headless or footless, but to have a middle and members, composed in fitting relation to each other and to the whole."
21 Stephen Halliwell, *Aristotle's Poetics* (University of Chicago Press, 1998). See also: Norman N. Holland, "Unity, Identity, Text, Self", *Publications of the Modern Language Association of America 90:5* (1975), 813–822.
22 Like in a detective story, the patient begins the therapeutic journey from the traces of the past that are found in the present, which lead him to the discovery of the havoc that lies in the past. The reader, like the therapist, copes with the ways in which the story is told (the "Syuzhet") and proceeds to deduce the chronological and causal order of events (the "Fabula") that lead from the past to the present. See: Peter Brooks, "Fictions of the Wolfman: Freud and Narrative Understanding", *Diacritics 9:1* (1979), 72–83; Jonathan

Culler, "Fabula and Syuzhet in the Analysis of Narrative", *Poetics Today 1:3* (1980), 27–37.

23 For more on this subject, see: Jacques Lacan and Jeffrey Mehlman, "Seminar on 'The Purloined Letter'", *Yale French Studies 48* (1972), 39–72; Harold T. Bloom, ed., *Defence and Resistance: Historical Perspectives and Current Concepts* (International Universities Press, 1985); Shoshana Felman, "On Reading Poetry: Reflections on the Limits and Possibilities of Psychoanalytic Approaches", in *The Literary Freud (Psychiatry and the Humanities 4)*, ed. Joseph H. Smith (Yale University Press, 1980), 119–148; Geoffrey H. Hartman, ed., *Psychoanalysis and the Question of the Text* (Johns Hopkins University Press, 1979); Ruth Nevo, *Shakespeare's Other Languages* (Routledge, [1987] 2021). For a comprehensive investigation of the transference between the reader and the author through the text's subconscious, see: Merav Roth, *A Psychoanalytic Perspective on Reading Literature: Reading the Reader* (Routledge, 2019).

24 Jean Laplanche and Jean-Bertrand Pontalis, *The Language of Psychoanalysis*, trans. Donald Nicholson Smith (Routledge, 1973), 103.

25 Sigmund Freud, "The Neuro-Psychoses of Defence", in *The Standard Edition of the Complete Psychological Works, Vol. 3: Early Psycho-Analytical Publications*, ed. and trans. James Strachey (Hogarth Press, 2001), 45–61; Sigmund Freud, "Jokes and Their Relation to the Unconscious", in *The Standard Edition, Vol. 8: Strachey* (Hogarth Press, 2001); Sigmund Freud, "Fragment of an Analysis of a Case of Hysteria, Three Essays on Sexuality and Other Works", in *The Standard Edition of the Complete Psychological Works of Sigmund Freud, Vol. 7, Strachey* (Hogarth Press, 2001); Sigmund Freud, "Inhibitions, Symptoms and Anxiety", in *The Standard Edition, Vol. 20, Strachey* (Hogarth Press, 2001); George E. Vaillant, "The Historical Origins and Future Potential of Sigmund Freud's Concept of the Mechanisms of Defence", *International Review of Psycho-Analysis 19:3* (1992), 5–50.

26 Nathan Alterman, "A Foreign Poem", in *Stars Outside* (Hakibbutz Hameuhad, 1938), 46-48 [Hebrew].

27 Sigmund Freud, "Remembering, Repeating, and Working-Through", in *The Standard Edition, Vol. 12: The Case of Schreber, Papers on Technique and Other Works, Strachey* (Hogarth Press, 2001), 145–157.

28 Matthew H. Erdelyi, *Psychoanalysis: Freud's Cognitive Psychology* (Freeman, 1985).

29 Helene Deutsch, "Discussion Remarks on a Developmental Approach to Problems of Acting Out", *Monographs of the American Academy of Child Psychiatry 1* (1966); Erdelyi, *Psychoanalysis*; Otto Fenichel, "Neurotic Acting Out", *Psychoanalytic Review 32:2* (1945), 197–206; Freud, "Remembering"; Phyllis Greenacre, "General Problems of Acting Out", *The Psychoanalytic Quarterly 19:4* (1950), 455–467; Dominick LaCapra, *History and Memory after Auschwitz* (Cornell University Press, 1998); Laplanche and Pontalis, *Language of Psychoanalysis*; Alex Holder and Joseph Sandler, *The Patient and the Analyst* (Maresfield Reprints, 1982).

30 Freud, "Remembering, Repeating, and Working Through", 150.

31 Freud, "Remembering, Repeating, and Working Through", 155.

32 Dominick LaCapra, "Representing the Holocaust: Reflections on the Historians' Debate", in Saul Friedländer, ed., *Probing the Limits of Representation* (Harvard University Press, 1992), 108–127; Laplanche and Pontalis, *Language of Psychoanalysis*.

33 Erdelyi, *Psychoanalysis*.

34 The concept of "aesthetic distance" is central to poetic language as defined by Bullough; see Edward Bullough, "Psychical Distance as a Factor in Art and an Aesthetic Principle", *British Journal of Psychology 5:2* (1912), 87–118. Aesthetic distance refers to the degree of emotional distance between the subject and the poetic work.

35 Hans W. Loewald, "On the Therapeutic Action of Psychoanalysis", *International Journal of Psychoanalysis 41* (1960), 16–33.

36 LaCapra, *History and Memory*, 20–21.
37 LaCapra, *History and Memory*, 20–21.
38 LaCapra, *History and Memory*, 20–21.
39 See Hephaestus's words to Thetis when asked to craft a shield for her son Achilles in the Iliad; Homer, *The Iliad*, trans. Peter Green (University of California Press, 2015), Book 18, 478–617.
40 Homer, *Iliad*.
41 Because I will be presenting texts that address personal traumatic experiences, the boundaries between the writer, the experience itself, and its representation in the poetic text are blurred. The same happens to the boundaries between the reader, who becomes a witness to this written experience, and the text.
42 Dudai, "Study of Poetic Devices".
43 This expression is taken from Hans Blumenberg, *Shipwreck with Spectator*, trans. Steven Rendall (MIT Press, 1996).
44 Dudai, "Study of Poetic Devices that Convey Restraint." This work was advised carried out under the advice of Prof. Reuven Tzur at Tel Aviv University, to whom I am extremely grateful for his insightful guidance and the deep influence he had on broadening my horizons beyond the literary field.
45 Aharon Appelfeld, *Searing Light* (Hakibbutz Hameuhad, 1980). [Hebrew]; Aharon Appelfeld, *The Man Who Never Stopped Sleeping*, trans. Jeffrey M. Green (Schocken Books, [2010] 2017).
46 Ka-Tzetnik, *The House of Dolls*, trans. Moshe M. Kohn (Simon and Schuster Inc., [1953] 1955).
47 Primo Levi, *If This Is a Man, The Truce*, trans. Stuart Woolf (Sphere Books LTD, [1958] 1987).
48 Blumenberg Hans, *Shipwreck with Spectator*, trans. Steven Rendall (MIT Press, 1996).

References

Agamben, Giorgio, *Remnants of Auschwitz: The Witness and the Archive* (Zone Books, 1999).

Alterman, Nathan, "A Foreign Poem", in *Stars Outside* (Hakibbutz Hameuhad, 1938), 46–48. [Hebrew].

Amir, Dana, *Bearing Witness to the Witness: A Psychoanalytic Perspective on Four Modes of Traumatic Testimony* (Routledge, 2018).

Appelfeld, Aharon, "Beyond Tragedy", in *First Person Essays* (World Zionist Organization, 1979), 49. [Hebrew].

Appelfeld, Aharon, *Searing Light* (Hakibbutz Hameuhad, 1980). [Hebrew].

Appelfeld, Aharon, *The Man Who Never Stopped Sleeping*, trans. Jeffrey M. Green (Schocken Books, [2010] 2017).

Blumenberg, Hans, *Shipwreck with Spectator*, trans. Steven Rendall (MIT Press, 1996).

Brooks, Peter, "Fictions of the Wolfman: Freud and Narrative Understanding", *Diacritics 9:1* (1979), 72–83.

Bullough, Edward, "Psychical Distance as a Factor in Art and an Aesthetic Principle", *British Journal of Psychology 5:2* (1912), 87–118.

Caruth, Cathy, ed., *Trauma: Explorations in Memory* (Johns Hopkins University Press, 1995).

Caruth, Cathy, *Unclaimed Experience* (Johns Hopkins University Press, 1996).

Celan Paul, *Selected Poems and Prose of Paul Celan*, trans. John Felstiner (Norton, [1955] 2001).

Culler, Jonathan, “Fabula and Syuzhet in the Analysis of Narrative”, *Poetics Today 1:3* (1980), 27–37.

Deutsch, Helene, “Discussion Remarks on a Developmental Approach to Problems of Acting Out”, *Monographs of the American Academy of Child Psychiatry 1* (1966), 144–172.

Dudai, Rina, “Study of Poetic Devices That Convey Restraint in the Charged Narrative Text” (MA Thesis, Tel Aviv, 1983), 7–18. [Hebrew].

Dudai, Rina, “Trauma in Translation: Crossing the Boundaries between Psychoanalysis and Film,”, *Projections 8:1* (2014), 41–60.

Erdelyi, Matthew H., *Psychoanalysis: Freud's Cognitive Psychology* (Freeman, 1985).

Felman, Shoshana, “On Reading Poetry: Reflections on the Limits and Possibilities of Psychoanalytic Approaches”, in Joseph H. Smith, ed., *The Literary Freud (Psychiatry and the Humanities 4)* (Yale University Press, 1980), 119–148

Felman, Shoshana and Laub, Dori, *Testimony: Crises of Witnessing in Literature, Psychoanalysis and History* (Routledge, 1992).

Fenichel, Otto, “Neurotic Acting Out”, *Psychoanalytic Review 32:2* (1945), 197–206.

Freud, Sigmund, “Fragment of an Analysis of a Case of Hysteria, Three Essays on Sexuality and Other Works”, in James Strachey ed. and trans., *The Standard Edition of the Complete Psychological Works of Sigmund Freud, Vol. 7, Strachey* (Hogarth Press, 2001).

Freud, Sigmund, “Inhibitions, Symptoms and Anxiety”, in James Strachey ed. and trans., *The Standard Edition, Vol. 20, Strachey* (Hogarth Press, 2001), 75–175.

Freud, Sigmund, “Jokes and Their Relation to the Unconscious,”, in James Strachey ed. and trans., *The Standard Edition of the Complete Psychological Works, Vol. 8: Strachey* (Hogarth Press, 2001), 1–236.

Freud, Sigmund, “Remembering, Repeating, and Working-Through”, in *The Standard Edition, Vol. 12: The Case of Schreber, Papers on Technique and Other Works, Strachey* (Hogarth Press, 2001), 145–156.

Freud, Sigmund, “The Neuro-Psychoses of Defence”, in James Strachey, ed. and trans., *The Standard Edition of the Complete Psychological Works, Vol. 3: Early Psycho-Analytical Publications* (Hogarth Press, 2001), 41–61.

Givoni, Michal, *The Ethics of Witnessing: A History of a Problem* (Hakibbutz Hameuchad, 2015). [Hebrew].

Goldberg, Amos, *Trauma in First Person: Diary Writing during the Holocaust* (Indiana University Press, 2017).

Greenacre, Phyllis, “General Problems of Acting Out”, *The Psychoanalytic Quarterly 19:4* (1950), 455–467.

Halliwell, Stephen, *Aristotle's Poetics* (University of Chicago Press, 1998).

Hartman, Geoffrey H., ed., *Psychoanalysis and the Question of the Text* (Johns Hopkins University Press, 1979).

Holder, Alex and Sandler, Joseph, *The Patient and the Analyst* (Maresfield Reprints, 1982).

Holland, Norman N., “Unity, Identity, Text, Self”, *Publications of the Modern Language Association of America 90:*5 (1975), 813–822.

Homer, *The Iliad*, trans. Peter Green (University of California Press, 2015), Book 18, 478–617.

Ka-Tzetnik, *The House of Dolls*, trans. Moshe M. Kohn (Simon and Schuster Inc., [1953] 1955).

Lacan, Jacques and Mehlman, Jeffrey, “Seminar on ‘The Purloined Letter’”, *Yale French Studies 48* (1972), 39–72.

LaCapra, Dominick, "Representing the Holocaust: Reflections on the Historians' Debate", in Saul Friedländer, ed., *Probing the Limits of Representation* (Harvard University Press, 1992), 108–127.

LaCapra, Dominick, *History and Memory after Auschwitz* (Cornell University Press, 1998).

LaCapra, Dominick, *Writing History, Writing Trauma* (John Hopkins University Press, 2001).

Laplanche, Jean and Pontalis, Jean-Bertrand, *The Language of Psychoanalysis*, trans. Donald Nicholson Smith (Routledge, 1973).

Levi, Primo, *If This Is a Man, The Truce*, trans. Stuart Woolf (Sphere Books LTD, [1958] 1987).

Loewald, Hans W., "On the Therapeutic Action of Psychoanalysis", *International Journal of Psychoanalysis 41* (1960), 16–33.

Lyotard, Jean-François, *The Differend: Phrases in Dispute*, trans. Georges Van Den Abbeele (University of Minnesota Press, 1988).

Lyotard, Jean-Francois and Ronan, John, *Anamnesis of the Visible* 2 (University of Nebraska Press, 1999). https://www.jstor.org/stable/20686094

Margalit, Avishai, *The Ethics of Memory* (Harvard University Press, 2002).

Nevo, Ruth, *Shakespeare's Other Languages* (Routledge, [1987] 2021).

Plato, *Phaedrus*, eds. Alexander Nehamas and Paul Woodruff (Hackett, 1995).

Roth, Merav, *A Psychoanalytic Perspective on Reading Literature: Reading the Reader* (Routledge, 2019).

Ullman, Chana, "Bearing Witness – Across the Barriers in Society and in the Clinic", *Psychoanalytic Dialogues 16:2* (2006), 181–198.

Vaillant, George E., "The Historical Origins and Future Potential of Sigmund Freud's Concept of the Mechanisms of Defence", *International Review of Psycho-Analysis 19:3* (1992), 5–50.

Part Two

Three Modes of Poetic Holocaust Testimony

Chapter 3

On Bodily Traumatic Memory in Aharon Appelfeld's *Searing Light*[1] and *The Man Who Never Stopped Sleeping*[2]

The traumatic event inscribed on Aharon Appelfeld's body can be glimpsed in his writings through his own mirroring shield, through his textual defense mechanisms, which are, in their turn, reflected in the various poetic devices he used in his writing. In this chapter, I investigate these textual mirroring shields, which enabled the writer to recount, throughout his oeuvre, what was engraved in his body.

Aharon Appelfeld, a Biography

Aharon (Ervin) Appelfeld was born in Jadova, a village near Czernowitz, then Romania, now Ukraine, on February 16, 1932, to a non-observant Jewish family. His father, an affluent man who had been educated in Vienna, worked on the automatization of flour mills. Both his maternal and paternal grandfathers were traditional Jews affiliated with the Hasidic courts of Sadigora and Vishnitz, respectively. While his parents spoke German, his grandparents used Yiddish. In spite of the generally assimilated atmosphere in his parental home, Jewishness trickled through, he recounted.[3] His mother was murdered at the beginning of the war when, in June 1940, Romania joined Nazi Germany and invaded Russia. Appelfeld was eight years old at the time.

The Jewish population of Czernowitz, including Appelfeld's family, were expelled and forced to walk to Transnistria, in southwest Ukraine, today's Moldova. Many perished on the way. The march took four months, until they reached an abandoned *kolkhoz* in Mohyliv-Podilskyi. At this point, the women and children were separated from the men. Appelfeld would not see his father again until 1957, when they were reunited in Israel.

Appelfeld escaped the camp and wandered through villages and forests, concealing his Jewish identity. At times he found shelter with Ukrainian farmers whose language he knew from overhearing the servants in his parents' home. Marginal people were living in the periphery of the villages: prostitutes and horse thieves

DOI: 10.4324/9781003403753-6

who could use the boy as a helper. They took him in without questions. Later, Appelfeld would say:

> Those war years were the most important years of my life. This was my elementary school, and also a bit of my high school, even though I was never enrolled in any such institution. I was in the forests, in the camps, the ghettos, all kinds of places… I learned from water, trees, animals, farmers, the people I met during the war, after the war. That was my school… which first shaped my reflexes to the world and my thoughts about the world… The war is my deepest basis, I never encountered anything like it anywhere.[4]

The Soviet army arrived in 1944. Meeting some Jews among the soldiers, Appelfeld joined them. With them, and along with the army, he moved via Romania and Bulgaria, from which, together with nine other Jewish boys, he fled to Yugoslavia and from there to Italy. Somewhere near Naples the boys were given food and shelter in a monastery – it was for the first time after a long period. This episode left a strong impression on Appelfeld: the silence, prayer, and church bells. Still, they left this place, too. They met a soldier who was enlisted in the Jewish Brigade under the British army, and he encouraged them to immigrate to pre-statehood Israel. They crossed the Mediterranean in the immigrant vessel "Hahagana" and landed in Palestine in 1946. Seized by the British Mandate authorities, the ship's passengers were jailed in Atlit – another camp on Appelfeld's long journey.

Toward the end of the year, the children were transferred to a Zionist youth village near Jerusalem. Appelfeld studied and worked there until Israel's war of independence in 1948. The children were transferred to the Mikveh Yisrael Agricultural School for their safety. Appelfeld was conscripted to the Israeli army in 1950 and completed his high school matriculation toward the end of his military service. During his time at the Hebrew University of Jerusalem, he studied Yiddish literature and became acquainted with the literary critic and scholar Dov Sadan, who became a formative figure for Appelfeld. Appelfeld first wrote poetry, then essays, only to move on to prose fiction in the late 1950s.[5] Appelfeld published scores of books until his death in 2018: collections of short stories, novellas, and collections of essays. Other works of his appeared in periodicals and have yet to be collected.[6]

Already with the publication in 1962 of his story "Berta" (in the collection *Smoke*),[7] Appelfeld began to be identified as a Holocaust author who was writing about "there" rather than "here." Years later, Appelfeld recalled that: thirty years later, Appelfeld recollected:

> From the moment I published my short story 'Berta', […] more than thirty years ago, they never stopped bothering me with questions about when I would write about life here in Israel […] Because I did not meet this request, over the years it turned into accusation and blame: He belongs there, he isn't one of us […] He's too much of a Jew, he's too detached from society […]trying to drag us

> back there. [...] There was a degree of arrogance, coming from the natives [...] a true conviction that everything began right here and what was not from here was destined to sink into oblivion.[8]

Appelfeld's attempts to have his first collection published were met with repeated rejection. Publishers wondered why his protagonists were so passive. Others asked how a young generation of Israelis was supposed to be raised on stories like this. When the short story collection *Smoke*[9] was finally published in 1962, critics commented that the protagonists were passive and unproductive.[10] Appelfeld, though, continued to turn to the faraway places in Europe he had left behind. In these formative years he found himself time and again being drawn back to seeds of memory related to orphanhood and loss. This became his mirror language: "Whenever I closed my eyes or picked up my pen I was back there."[11]

The story of Appelfeld's life is very different from his local, Israeli-born coevals. This is what he said in an interview with Yigal Schwartz:

> I wanted somehow to think of myself like the literary heroes of those days: tall, blond, blue eyes. That was the ideal figure they presented me with. [...] But I also felt something else, which I couldn't explain to myself at the time.[12]

It is this "something else" that lifted Appelfeld out of the mainstream of Hebrew literature. His plots were unlike those of the Israeli Sabra; his landscape was not Israel, and the kind of lives that dominate his books are not exactly like those of this country's pioneering settlement.[13]

Appelfeld's Hebrew antecedents were S.Y. Agnon, Dov Sadan, and the Yiddish author Leib Rochman, who treated him like a son. Agnon offered Appelfeld a model of writing that allowed him to relate to his past: the Jewish, and not the Israeli, past. The same was the case with Sadan, who had started his career at the Hebrew University of Jerusalem, teaching Yiddish, and endorsed Appelfeld's way of reconnecting with Jewish culture.[14] Appelfeld called Sadan "the man with the little torchlight." He rekindled Appelfeld's feelings for his ravaged and forgotten home.[15] It was the encounter with these two men that restored young Appelfeld to himself, to his culture of origin, and to the experience of the Jewish diaspora, which did not feature significantly in Israeli culture at that time. Appelfeld's relationship with Rochman, fourteen years his senior, was extremely close.[16] It was from him he derived the religious sentiment infusing his work, and it was Rochman who inspired the quiet howl in Appelfeld's non-pathetic writing. Rochman was the person who, during years of darkness and concealment, held out his hand and lifted him up.[17]

Style: Restraint and Subtlety

Until the 1990s, when he published *The Iron Tracks*,[18] *The Ice Mine*,[19] and *The Story of a Life*,[20] Appelfeld chose only to suggest the flames but not to be burned or consumed by them. He achieves this by making quiet, subtle, and restrained contact with what came before the traumatic experience and what followed it. At this stage he did not directly engage with it. He did not touch the terrible things that happened between 1939 and 1946. He cut out the most terrible of all. Appelfeld exposed the approaching catastrophe before the war broke out and the traces of terror following it. This choice of narrative temporality reflects an attempt to reduce, as much as possible, human description and artistic form. The most terrible time remained unvoiced until the 1990s.

Following the publication, in the early 1960s, of Appelfeld's first book, *Smoke*, the poet Uri Zvi Greenberg told Appelfeld he considered his writing an "expression reined in," while making light of critics' description of it as "restrained writing." "What is 'restraint'?" he mocked. "If you have something to say, then say it, and say it loud and clear," demanding him to deliver his message loud and clear. One cannot speak of great catastrophes in whispers, he explained.[21] But pathos and big words being far from Appelfeld's sensibility and writing style, he preferred subtle language and observation.[22]

Appelfeld's restraint captivated reviewers. In his book *Open Notebook: Discussions of Current Israeli Fiction*,[23] Dan Miron wrote that the narrator in Appelfeld's stories is a mature figure who manages to represent the psychological and moral impact of the Holocaust experience in a responsible and subtle manner.[24] Gershon Shaked, in his *A New Wave in Hebrew Fiction*,[25] believed that the choice to write about the Holocaust inaugurated a new direction for Hebrew literature. He wrote that even though Appelfeld's subject matter was emotionally charged, and the characters that peopled his stories were small-time victims caught up in a terrifying, nightmarish reality full of death, the author managed to steer clear of pathos by using a restrained and very personal style.[26] In his article *Appelfeld's Affinity with Kafka*, Hillel Barzel argues that "In Appelfeld, compassion trades places with subtlety. The language describing absolute evil is soft and poetic [...] Things are whispered as if they were uttered voicelessly."[27] These critics and others[28] use near-identical terms when discussing Appelfeld's style. In 1983, Appelfeld was awarded the Israel Prize, the country's most prestigious prize for cultural achievement. In its recommendations the board of judges wrote that Appelfeld's singular portrayal of the Jewish individual both before and after the Holocaust rendered him in a restrained, subtle and formally stylistic manner.

As suggested, however, not all readers felt as appreciative of Appelfeld's restraint. Some saw it as a stylistic failure, while others argued that his style was more charged than initially met the eye,[29] while Hever, Oppenheimer, and Alon[30] did not consider Appelfeld a restrained writer in the first place. In their view, critics failed to note the traumatic acting-out his works constitute, the traces of trauma they carry – something that, far from being restrained, makes these works charged texts. For Hever, most of the criticism and research has been misled by Appelfeld's linguistic minimalism, something about which Appelfeld himself said the following: "I try to be spare with words in order to make feeling and thought more visible."[31]

Schwartz is the critic who has done the most profound research of Appelfeld's oeuvre.[32] Within that broad perspective he addresses the critics' blind spot: A consensus gradually evolved about the writer describing his Holocaust experience in a lyrical mode, his stories constituting a subtle artistic experience of sublimation concerning the trauma of the Holocaust.[33] Schwartz expands the discussion in hopes of releasing Appelfeld from this post-traumatic template. The Holocaust is only one station on Appelfeld's way, which also covered the Austro-Hungarian empire period and – in the third phase of his writing – an effort to join the national-tribal Zionist narrative.[34]

My point of departure in this chapter is not a developmental-historical one. I intend to show that the date of composition and the nature of the historical period during which it was written do not matter in the case of Appelfeld's work. The traumatic core, the "toxic, radioactive waste"[35] that affects his subject matter and his singular style, has consistently dictated the nature of his writing. Confined to this experience, Appelfeld's writing keeps turning around it, almost unable to find release. Something profound, beyond time and space, in Appelfeld's writing produces poetic testimony, and it is related to his sense of obligation to testify to what shaped and defined his world: his experience of the Holocaust. What enabled him to write such testimony, I believe, is the use of a poetic textual mechanism that contains the pathetic and sentimental elements immanent in the traumatic thematic, creating an impression of restraint and subtlety, which prevents the text's collapse.

My main question is whether Appelfeld's stylistic imprint and his quiet restraint are a formal device the writer used to overcome the pathetic fallacy[36] or, alternatively, a textual defense mechanism required by the traumatic nature of his subject matter.[37] I will be considering this with reference to his novels *Searing Light* and *The Man Who Never Stopped Sleeping*.

Restraint in *Searing Light*

The novel *Searing Light* (1980) looks at the early stages of rehabilitation of children who have recently arrived from Europe; it is a description of adolescent Holocaust survivors' attempt to adjust to everyday life in a Zionist agricultural-residential school in Eretz Israel, i.e., mandatory Palestine. An abyss, however, is threatening just beyond daily routine: chaos is imminent once the layer of banality is removed. Terrible things happen in the course of the novel: both Bloch and the housemother go crazy; Blum commits suicide; Regina becomes a victim of gang rape; Mindro and Blanca go missing; Laufer, Druck, and other boys are expelled; Mintz becomes disabled, and the other boys continuously harass each other. In addition, using materials related to the period before the Holocaust, Appelfeld portrays a state of fragmentation there too, not directly tied to the Holocaust. This is rendered through an examination of the small family where the father turns out to have intended to leave his family before the outbreak of the war (Chapter 14).

Thematically speaking, Appelfeld documents a horrific exposure to a chaotic reality that does not admit any sense or meaning. The novel's central axis is formed by the characters' senseless drifting from one place to another. Each chapter offers another perspective on the same, never-resolved theme, namely the world in chaos.

Appelfeld's decision to reject pathos forces him to look for other devices. While constructing a pathetic and dramatic world, he chooses to represent it by means of restraint and subtlety. He does not remove or neutralize the emotional charge of his materials. He leads his reader to the very cusp of emotional release and then brings to bear a system of devices that produce restraint, abruptly changing the organization of the charged materials.

Four types of devices construct this sense of textual restraint: minimization, blunting, fragmentation, and equivalence.[38] The first device, *minimization*, helps to block the charged material or communicate it in an incomplete, limited manner. This leads to gaps in the textual material in which the charged subject matter is concealed or encoded. When Appelfeld uses *blunting*, he makes his material obscure and blurred. Next, the *dissociative* device presents contents in a fragmentary manner and out of context. What these three devices have in common is that they suspend the transition between perception and conceptualization or judgment by focusing attention on the process of perception as such. This dwelling on the textual material rather than on its content shifts the center of gravity from subject matter to its organization. Now the charged subject matter is not exposed as intensively focused substance but is enfolded and encoded in complex and obscure expressions. The fourth and final device, *equivalence*, ensures that all components of the text are ascribed equal importance. This rejection of priorities or hierarchies enables the author to insert and encode threatening content into less threatening, more banal, everyday ones.

It is this system of restraining devices that, I believe, controls the text and regulates the emotional intensities of the subject matter. The way these devices are employed – their location in the text, the intensity of their deployment – may at times clash with other directions into which the text also pulls. The outcome is a tense constellation, carrying a potent emotional tendency that is blocked just before its climax.[39] Below I present an analysis of these devices at work at different textual levels: lexical, syntactic, figurative, and structural.

The Device of Minimization

This device involves the blockage of information that was meant to be conveyed, and it occurs on different levels of the narrative: the lexical, syntactic, figurative, and structural.

Minimization on the Lexical Level

One way by which reduction produces a sense of missing information occurs through the use of suggestion or *deixis*. According to Lyons, expressions of this kind are, for instance "this," "that," "here," or "there" – words pointing at a place, object, person, or event in a context of concrete and specific time and place.[40] The perspective of the one who uses these words is the zero point of reference;

observation is situated in the speaker without taking into account where the other is in relation to him or her.[41] The speaker uses these terms to indicate the spatial area in which the object of observation can be found. Appelfeld uses suggestive terms to draw attention to the spatial background while suppressing and concealing the object itself. Often this leads to an immediately concrete and authentic effect, resulting from the assumption that the object of observation is within the visual range and within the physical reach of both narrator and readers. But while using this effect, Appelfeld empties it of meaning. Instead of drawing attention to the object, deixis is fully directed at the spatial background, which constitutes a kind of empty frame, from which the main thing, the object, is missing.

I call this Appelfeld's "hollow deixis." In this deployment of minimization, a clash occurs between the expectation of a very specific kind of information, on one hand, while major information is being withheld, on the other – either by hiding it or by dealing, instead, with unimportant background material. Here is an example: "Mintz raised both his arms and said: 'That's it. That's it.'"[42] In another example, from Chapter 1 of *Searing Light*: "Mintz did not wait, he acted. Who knows what he did, Bloch did not yell. Morning revealed that we were moles."[43] Mintz is about to come up with Bloch's verdict. The reader does not know what act on Bloch's part the verdict is about and what Mintz has decided. "This is it" allows one to refer to an extremely dramatic, concrete, and loaded event while at the same time keeping it unnamed, encoded, and implicit.

Deixis supports the device of reduction. Indeed, the reader has no access to the important, main information until the end of the chapter and until the end of the novel, even though it seems to be almost within view.

While the novel's dominant subject is how people cope with their experience of the Holocaust, it very rarely refers to past events. Events occurring in the narrative present, however, are often rendered in a language that echoes images from the Holocaust. These expressions function like code words, serving to linguistically "shift" readers from the present into the past and back again, thus producing the threatening connection. For instance:

> And still in shock, we were already on our way, taken along. A pickup loaded with sacks collected us [...] Now the place was full. Clothes were piled up by the windows. [...] 'So, when do they go?' 'Soon' said the official, 'They're organizing a transport.' And that's how he handed us over. [..] Lights of day showed in the shacks' windows reminding the heart of the jolting in locked night train carriages. [...] The official stood in the door opening, indignant. [...] To us he said: 'Why don't you go to the container. They're handing out soup for free. [...] The transport won't leave all that soon' [...].[44]

This passage appears in the first part of *Searing Light*, and recounts the boys' time in southern Italy. Lonely and destitute, they wander aimlessly. Thus, they end up in a refugee camp, where the Jewish Agency is organizing a group of children to travel to Eretz Israel, the Zionist settlement in Palestine. Through the references to reality that are in tune with the language describing this event, code words can be glimpsed. Terms like "camp," "transport," "block," soup distribution, or "locked night train carriages" resurrect the nightmarish world of the Holocaust. Not many words are needed. The way that these words are being used and inflected in the description of everyday reality makes it clear how powerful the trap of trauma is. Introducing these materials into the description of immigration to Eretz Israel has more than a hint of the grotesque – which is projected onto what for Appelfeld's average reader is a major value: immigration to (pre-state) Israel – here however by way of another transport.

Another, even bolder instance appears in the interrogation of the Laufer and Druck boys by the unmarried woman at the educational institution where they have been put up:

> Then, trembling, Druck, was taken to the office. To the unmarried woman's many questions he did confess that he had caressed Ventura's legs, but it had been with her consent, in exchange for cigarettes and sweets. The unmarried woman asked: 'What did you come here for, do you know?'
>
> 'Of course I know,' said Druck, his distress abated, 'To work the land'. 'And what else?'
>
> 'To love our homeland?'
>
> 'And what else?'
>
> 'To remember the Holocaust.'
>
> 'And you, what did you do.'
>
> 'I caressed Ventura's legs.'
>
> Now all that remained was to enquire after some secret details. About the ghetto, about the camp, and about the terrible transport which had separated him and his parents. Druck recounted while pulling at the button on his jacket. Unable to tolerate the touch, the unmarried woman quickly told him off. For a moment, her comment embarrassed him. But he went on. The unmarried woman though had run out of patience and said 'That's it.' [...]
>
> The judgment was executed on the following day [...] Druck was afraid this time they would really punish him, move him inland [...] It was true, just then there were rumors of grim institutions, further into the land, among the remote, exposed hills, which wouldn't let you out more than once a month, on organized trips. 'They'll send me away, they'll send me away,' he sobbed [...]
>
> There were no signs of expulsion but his fears did not subside. Again, he huddled by the old rucksacks. His face wore a worried expression, like during the war when they were waiting for a transport.
>
> 'Don't worry so much about yourself,' Laufer tormented him.
>
> [...]
>
> 'So, imagine you're in the camp. You can do that.'
>
> 'What do you mean? I've been in seven camps. I remember their names.'
>
> 'So, if you were in seven of them, you won't mind one more.'[45]

This quote exemplifies the power of scaled-down expression. Visual fragments taken from dramatic situations like separation, expulsion, and drifting form the tip of the iceberg gradually coming into view in the narrative present. Suggested interactions between present and past are not in one direction only. Events in the here and now raise images from the past, but these fragments subsequently become stuck back in the present, which they overshadow. The powerfully ironic parallel in Laufer's following words, "So if you were in seven of them, you won't mind one more,"[46] opens out into a multi-directional nightmarish world which locks the characters in a cycle of terror. The Holocaust experience leaks into the present, leaving these characters with no way out.[47]

This heavy feeling, conveyed in a loud whisper, resonates at the end of the novel. *Searing Light* concludes with the real situation of military enlistment on the eve of Israel's war of independence – the boys are described as they climb into a truck:

> The hugely powerful wish that had been pounding within us from that morning was running empty. A dark tiredness held us together close by the walls. Like in past times, on small train stations, all we wanted was to close our eyes, surrender to slumber.
>
> The truck arrived late at night. The driver, coming out of the cabin, called out angrily: 'Where are they? Where?' The angry shouting tore us from sleep, all at once. The driver pulled the stubborn hook and the door slammed. As in sleep, no need for words. One after the other, the bodies poured into the cargo bed.[48]

It is hard to avoid the comparison here, between actively joining the army to fight in the war of independence, and the victim's passive conveyance to yet another concentration camp. The comparison casts a tragic light onto the military mobilization.

Minimization on the Syntactic Level

A prominent stylistic feature is Appelfeld's use of simple sentences. Sentences tend to be short, even very short. Sometimes they are incomplete. At other times they don't connect, and the writing falters. Each sentence stands alone, in isolation, surrounded by silence. Here is an example:

> But we don't care. When evening approaches, we go to the beach, to get into the water, immerse ourselves for a bit in the surrounding distraction. Traders, smugglers, a host of colors and drinks. Some temporary buildings have already turned permanent. Plenty of ice cream.[49]

This passage offers a description consisting of crumbling images, which, taken together, suggest an evening on a beach. This assemblage of parts, in the absence of a unifying frame, has an effect of reduction or minimalism, but also of gaps. Here is another example:

> It turns out he never met my father face to face.
> How could he have reached him.
> My father was in the capital, he in the provinces.

The newspapers in the capital would return his manuscripts.
He was forced to publish in the godforsaken provincial press.
All agreed his criticism was serious.
But over there in the capital they didn't bother responding.
It would have encouraged him, had there been a response from the capital.
Not sure if he'd ever write again.[50]

Here the speaker receives some indirect information about his father from Shtrum, a literary critic, who was in touch with his father before the war. The text suggests rejection and great vulnerability, even if much time has passed since then. The knowledge that he was probably saved because his reviews were not accepted in the capital, since if he had moved there, he would certainly have died, does not offer any relief or solace. The sense of rejection and offense outweighs any possible happiness about staying alive. The sorrow, pain, and vulnerability are communicated in short, staccato sentences. They are merely informative and maintain a reticent restraint. Such relevant and useful information as passes hands constitutes traces of the disaster, but it is a disaster that has remained unarticulated.

Figurative Minimization

In the course of time, Appelfeld sheds more and more of the ballast of figurative language, increasingly confronting difficult issues by means of direct, sparse language. In an interview with Avraham Balaban, Appelfeld mentioned that this lessening use of metaphor was intended: "My development is from metaphoric expression to a more direct mode [...] I tried to keep metaphor to a minimum."[51] Indeed, metaphor appeared much less emphatically, its main function remaining to render a condensed atmosphere, unfocused, resonating psychological states, or an incomplete representation of a lost world.

Searing Light hardly ever reports directly on inner reflections, dreams, fantasies, or hallucinations. The characters' mental life, which takes place below the surface, can be gathered from shreds of conversation, from the unfolding events, and from landscape descriptions. These descriptions of the landscape out there in the world constitute a kind of reflection or projection of the inner, human landscapes which the work does not yield. Landscapes offer a compensatory, camouflaged peeping hole into protagonists' inner worlds. Here are some random illustrations: "One after the other, shutters closed over windows, darkness pressing itself into the spaces between houses,"[52] "[...] but already I was a long way away from the house, into the night, into the thirst-quenching blue that covered me, broad and transparent like the double wings of a blue hornet,"[53] or "Leftover heat and the shades of night spread like a huge net."[54] It is easy to see that these landscape descriptions serve as illustrations of an oppressive inner experience.

In these landscape descriptions figurative language is deployed at its most extensive, through metaphor, metonymy, and synecdoche. Metonymy and synecdoche render concrete, albeit in a partial manner, worlds that no longer exist. This figurative tool represents two elements that are absent from the narrative present: the reality of the Holocaust (a negative reality which the characters try to shed) and that of home and childhood (a positive reality for which the characters yearn).

The Holocaust as a negative essence without direct representation in the text may show itself in the course of a description of everyday life in the present and slip in as an apparently innocent, trivial detail, then assume frightening meaning, exposing what was buried under the debris. This is what happens in Chapter 15, the boys' life in the residential school: "Peals of laughter would belch out into the night as from chimneys."[55] In the everyday context, we see an active image, lively and noisy: noise that is audible outside the boys' dormitories at night. But through the figurative phrase, the boys' shouts come to be likened to smoke belching from chimneys. The shift to the seemingly naive detail of the chimneys in the middle of a description of the jolly atmosphere in the residential school introduces tension and an ominous feeling once its extra-textual associations come into play associations with extermination. This figurative detail becomes an encoded sign referring to everything related to the horrific reality. The metonymy here paints the laughter and shouting in a hue that no longer has anything in common with joy. And now that the associative process has been set into motion, with the chimneys functioning as a metonymic vehicle taking the reader to the Holocaust, other elements, which so far did not make themselves very manifest, take an active role in this image, like the combination of shouting and laughing and the transposition of voice (shouts) into image (smoke belching out and up from the chimneys). Now the text no longer merely refers to the boys' mischievous laughter but invokes a shout that goes up in smoke, a kind of loud silence. Once the image becomes filled with the perspective of what the metonym represents, it ties into the broader context of annihilation and extinction.

The memory of home and childhood, unlike that of the Holocaust, which briefly surges at unexpected moments, hovers throughout the entire text as a fantasy which has no direct representation. A detailed examination of Chapter 1 of *Searing Light* bears out how minimal means render traces of the existence of an entire world that perished forever.

Chapter 1 offers a description of the four boys, Holocaust refugees, wandering along the coast of southern Italy. They drift aimlessly until at some point they notice a building in the far distance: "The distant, nice-looking structure with its two sloping roofs was beckoning and reminded of warmth, steaming milk, and bread just coming out of the oven."[56] This sets into motion a dynamic that is wholly dominated by the attempt to approach the building. The structure – a concrete object which stands out against the sandy background of the beach – is described in terms that exceed the merely functional. The building has a magical pull on the boys, resurrecting images they associate with home. Even though they see the structure from a distance, vaguely, they complete the image into a shape they have been trying to repress for years. These fragments of an image – the structure eventually proves to be a neglected, abandoned shed, a disused military depot – synecdochally remind them of everything they have lost and which, now, they hallucinate, they might find again. In their imagination, the boys complete their vision of the structure with its sloping roofs, turning it into a pastoral home that rouses the senses which have been suppressed.

This image of derelict building instigates three main feelings in the boys, feelings associated with a sense of the safe home: "hot milk," "hotbread," "hot oven." Memories are embodied in concrete imagery related to the senses: vision, hearing, and the sense of warmth – all of which correlate with body memories, in this case, memories that trigger a psychological experience of security and stability. As the boys approach the building, this feeling only intensifies, to the point of acquiring a kind of religious, ecstatic overtone, as though the boys are being, in a way, miraculously drawn toward their destiny.

The boys' disappointment is not merely about the shoddy, deserted building they eventually encounter: it is mainly about the hidden dreams and desires which were triggered by this vision. Emotion, repressed for years, has briefly erupted, passing through all the defensive layers of reason, prompting their most archaic yearnings for a warm and safe home. The boys' intense, irrational behavior makes sense against the background of this metonymic effect of the abandoned depot on their mental reality, their desires, and their yearnings. Once their mistake becomes devastatingly clear, violence erupts as a wild, archaic need to wipe out what happened. Their enchantment with the building is tied up with their deep need to fill the lacuna of their orphanhood. The building caused their pangs for a warm and secure home to rise to the surface, their need for a lost safe world: "The magical building was resting stably and squarely on the horizon, tempting us."[57] The outburst of violence on realizing their error indicates, more than anything, how deprived they are. The red-tiled building forced the boys to rush after a replacement of their lost paradise – then to confront the deceptive nature of the trigger and be driven to violence or madness. Bloch, who did go crazy, internalized this miraculous yearning, only to find himself cut off from the world.

Structural Minimization

Reduction in communicated information leads to implicit, and eventually to blockage of important information in the description of dramatic events on the level of plot. One example relates to the story about Blum in Chapter 13. Information here is communicated by relegating it to a less important part of the plot – as if it were background material – and by a reduction, to the point of removal, of dramatic details. The chapter describes Blum and how he copes with the loss of his family; it takes off with the moment Blum starts spiraling down to devastation. Time and again the narrative dwells on the boy's character, which builds up a tense expectation of an approaching dramatic event:

> Little Blum, fat little Blum [...] started writing letters to his mother [...] Little Blum knew his mother was no longer alive, the street where he was born had been wiped from the face of the earth, and yet he wrote, not only that: he also sent.[58]

There turns out to be a considerable difference between the boy Blum and the other boys, who are immersed in their reveling: "And that's how we got ourselves, to be honest, disconnected from him. The cut was easy and painless."[59] At this point, with the background sufficiently substantial, the tragic tip of the iceberg can be glimpsed: "And while everything means summer, oblivion and foreign rash on a youthful body, Bloom disappears."[60] Blum, whose name promises blossoming, wilts and expires while nature blooms. His disappearance and the subsequent search for him grow more intense as time goes by. The mood is extremely charged emotionally, feelings that erupt in the encounter with the tradesmen and then again subside at the boys' defeated return to school in the morning: "Morning terror came upon us, suddenly, as if we were naked."[61] The climax everybody has been waiting for does not happen. A tense, helpless waiting sets in, rather, which will eventually harden and become inaccessible.

Yet once again, it is this hardening that is followed by tidings that vaguely suggest an answer: "A boy was floating on the sea, he looked like Blum. The sea must have cast him up."[62] The delayed climax, by this point, has accumulated power. This derives from both the subject matter and the narrative structure and mood, all of which are now replete with pathetic elements. Here, however, the story comes to a halt, unresolved with no closure:

> The man announced his bitter news and stood. [...] Because no one asked any more, not even the janitor, he turned his head like one grown used to thanklessness and moved aside, where the back door opened out on the sea.[63]

In a more conventional narrative, this would be the moment of resolution, now that the dramatic climax has been reached. This story, however, grinds to a halt and is left unresolved. Expected details about what happened fail to materialize, and the action ends without closure or a stable conclusion. The man who brought the tidings hastily leaves the stage, and the description is dominated by his offense at his words being ignored.

This episode is narrated in such a way that most of the information concerns the background to the plot's main event while keeping the main information concealed. This is how Appelfeld contrives to take his story all the way to the limit of pathos without getting caught up in it.

The Device of Blurring

This mode of indistinctness blurs and scatters materials through the text to represent the traumatic subject matter, if at all it is represented, in a highly attenuated form. This blunting, blurring, and scattering dulls the material by presenting it so that it is harder to perceive. There are several ways in which the text operationalizes this blurring device: on the syntactic as well as on the figurative and the structural levels.

Syntactic Blurring

In a fictional narrative some parts of the recounted events are marked as being of greater import than others; it is these parts that constitute the front stage of the narrative. The other, less major events come to form the background, assisting the reader to evaluate and orient themselves in relation to the main events.[64] One tactic Appelfeld uses to diminish and modify the charged nature of his materials is by unsettling the relations between foreground and background. What should have been right at the front of the plot thematically speaking – people's way of coping with the memory of their Holocaust experience – is pushed into the sidelines and lost in the background. While the novel's main scene describes minor, banal everyday events, blended in with them are harsh events like suicide, rape, and expulsion.

This inversion between foreground and background can be variously seen at work in the novel. Here are some examples of the level of language:

> When the janitor learned that his entire family, his two sisters, elder brothers, and his mother, had all been killed and were no longer alive – he donned the battledress and headed for the cowshed with large and measured strides. [...] And as though nothing had happened, he distributed fodder and filled the water trough. [...] Not one superfluous movement the janitor made. From one place to the next his hands hurried and within a short time the space was clean and washed.[65]

This is how Chapter 16 opens. It is exactly the part of the sentence that is syntactically the least dominant, the subordinate clause, which is the emotionally most charged. And, conversely, the part of the sentence describing routine everyday activity appears in the syntactically dominant main clause. The encounter between what should have been in the forefront and what actually is in that position creates a double dissonance: The intensity of terror is, on the one hand, attenuated when it appears disguised as ongoing routine activity, while the clash, on the other hand, between the two elements of the sentence intensifies what has not been expressed directly: "If he had found any point in my favor I would definitely have stayed in Vienna, roamed the streets, sat in the cafes, and ended up being killed like everyone else."[66]

As part of a modal sentence, "if," the sentence's most important semantic information is planted at its very end: "If he had found any point in my favor I would definitely have stayed in Vienna, roamed the streets, sat in the cafes, and ended up being killed like everyone else." The resulting subtle irony is produced by the syntactic position of the information, which marks it as equivalent to the previous units of information due to the deployment of the conjunction "and." The conjunction, which presents equivalence, forces readers to take in the strolling in the streets, spending time in cafés, and being destroyed along with everyone else – all with a similar degree of attention. This is how the threatening issue is conveyed in a subordinate manner. The semantically major event appears in a syntactically reductive position. It is by means of this inversion in the hierarchical relations among units of information and the clash between what is considered foreground and background material, respectively, that the terror is rerouted to "neutral," and "protected" foci.

Figurative Blurring

This is a form of blurring resulting from blunting textual materials, enabling the author to describe processes as they unfold, before they take definite shape. This discursive blunting or blurring gets in the way of an immediate passage from sensory contact to a conceptual judgment and evaluation by suspending attention and holding it focused on the reception of the object of observation rather than on its evaluation. This causes the represented experience to be felt as saturated and compressed,[67] yet unconceptualized. The receiver is aware of the concept's components but not of the concept itself. The information is blurred through the mixing of discursive domains – which is mainly achieved by the use of figurative language, which includes displacement from one discursive domain to another. Below I offer some illustrations, distinguishing between three types of figurative use: (1) Mixed domains between one sensory faculty and another, synesthesia, (2) mixed domains between an object with a well-defined form and an object lacking a well-defined form; (3) mixed domains between one object (a person) and another (animal, plant, or inanimate).

Discursive Mixing between One Sensory Faculty and Another

Example:

> Darkness flowed in through the mesh screen and filled the room with silence.[68]

Here blurring is achieved by the use of synesthesia. This is a psychological state in which two or more senses are experienced, while only one of them is actually activated. Research identifies it in descriptions where one sense experience is represented in terms of another. For instance, a sound might be attributed a color, a color might be associated with a smell, or a smell might be linked with a sound, and so on.[69] Synesthesia is the capacity to register correspondence between senses so that one sense will be perceived by means of the other. It is a type of very primitive metaphoric expression which elicits a subject's emotion without accompanying conceptual understanding.[70]

In the synesthetic description above we witness a visual motion of no-light/darkness entering a room and filling it with no-sound/silence. The image is very sensual, substituting, as it does, something that is meant to be perceived by one sense – vision – with something that comes under the sense of hearing. But this particular instance of synesthesia occurs in a perceptual condition of absence. Absence of light – darkness – transforms into absence of sound – silence. And in addition, absence as a quality shared by both light and sound is perceived as a movement whereby space (the room) becomes filled, directed from the outside in. This leaves the reader with a representation of reality whose components come together and fall apart at one and the same time. The movement that "fills" the lacuna, which is meant to be perceived by mixing senses – a transfer of movement from one sense (vision) to another (hearing) – registers and fails to register simultaneously. The structure exists. There is movement (from the outside in), there's space (the room), and there is an act of filling. But what should have been at the forefront of the filling movement, the content of the action, is absence itself: the absence of light and the absence of voice. What has been constructed perceptually comes apart conceptually. The perception of absence can only be achieved on the structural level.

Discursive Mixing between an Object with Well-Defined Form and an Object Lacking Well-Defined Form

Example:

> That night, a heavy sleep descended upon the boys. Not a sound was heard. In the dully lit bathrooms, the faucets, as though measuring the silence, produced a slow drip.[71]

A very common feature of this type of mixed discourse involves a gradual blurring of an object with a well-defined form, whose place then is taken over by an object that lacks a well-defined form. The result is a description that seeks to put words to a pre-conceptual reality. This paradox is the outcome of the text's persistent effort to represent reality at a low level of organization and of maximum concreteness, while avoiding generalizations or abstraction. More than seeking to offer clear, transparent, and explicit information, it creates a condensed atmosphere. This atmosphere is achieved by using semantic components that share meaning but that belong to different discursive domains. This produces an effect of an unnamable reality, which is felt as intense, saturated, and compressed.

In the example, we are presented with a concrete image of sparsely illuminated toilets at night; there is not a living soul in this place, and the faucets are dripping, slowly and steadily. The accompanying image compares this dripping to a measure of silence. The space in between one drop falling and the next becomes a quantitative means of measuring silence. When dripping taps are observed conventionally, the taps will occupy the foreground, and the spaces between one drop and the next, the background. The figurative representation, however, turns perception upside down: now the foreground is no longer made up by the drops but by the intervals between them. The drops are perceived both visually and through the sound they make reaching the end of their trajectory. The metaphor shifts from vision to sound by amplifying the auditory elements at the expense of the visual. Thus, once more, the essence of absence is grasped through the transfer from vision to absence of sound to silence.

Another example: "[...] the darkness condensed itself between houses."[72] A similar principle is at work in this illustration. In the conventional mode the houses – the distinct form – will be perceived as foreground, and the formless dark as background. Here, however, things have changed positions, and as part of the cumulative process of movement, "condensed itself," darkness gains power and moves into the foreground, with the houses functioning as background. The non-distinct, non-embodied element thus comes to dominate the image, thereby increasing the impression of blurred domains and indistinction.

Example:

> Nights would fall warm and dark, as if crafted from black down.[73]

Here the object of observation and the modes of reception combine to highlight a state of indistinctness. By means of the adjectives "warm," "dark," and "black down," Appelfeld represents an intense and profound sensation of material expanding in an attempt to touch the object of observation prior to its having assumed form. The chosen senses, too, confirm this. Warmth is perceived by means of the thermic sense, which is considered primitive among the senses. Down registers via touch, which like thermic perception features low on the sensory scale. The warm and dark nights are perceived by means of senses whose level of conscious organization is low.

Example:

> Night erased the paths and we cast our way through the low darkness heading towards the lonely shack.[74]

If we want to paraphrase this figurative expression, we might say: "The night, like rain, erased the paths, and the boys plodded through the darkness as through mud." Contact with the darkness feels thick and sticky like mud. The intangibility of the dark takes on a concrete dimension; it can now be felt. The thematic subject suggested by this type of figurative choice is a sense of losing one's way: the erased paths and the pervasive dark are the only things perceived with certainty. Indistinctness comes to dominate representation.

Discursive Mixing between One Object (a Person) and Another (Animal, Plant, or Inanimate)

Metaphor, imagery, metonymy, personification, and projection are all common literary practices, and in this sense Appelfeld's novel is not singular. Still, arguably, Appelfeld's minimal use of figurative language supports the principle of indistinction because it allows the insertion of one discursive domain into another, blurring their boundaries. Another major device the novel uses is the insertion of the inanimate into the realm of plants, of plants into that of animals, and of animals into the human domain, and vice versa. While the inanimate environment undergoes animation, in parallel, the living soul is removed from the human realm. Images used in descriptions of humans evolve in the following direction: from the animal domain, at the beginning of the novel, via images and metaphors based on the vegetable domain, toward images and metaphors related to inanimate objects.

Here are some examples from the animal domain:

> The entire length of her acted like an animal returning to the stables.
>
> (Chapter 5)

> You drive me crazy.... Because you attach yourself to me like a leech.
>
> (Chapter 9)

> Like bad animals we'd lay in wait for him at the door.
>
> (Chapter 13)

And some from the vegetable domain:

> At times we would find him planted within himself.
>
> (Chapter 15)

> The little discovery immediately sprouted a wan smile of gratitude on the janitor's face.
>
> (Chapter 15)

And also some illustrations from the domain of inanimate objects:

> The driver maneuvered the pickup close to the door, and together they lifted the load on a broad and sloping plank.
>
> (Chapter 15; [the word "load" here refers to Yuko' body, wounded by the janitor's blows.])

> The bodies poured, one after the other, into the crate.
>
> (Chapter 17; [referring to the enlisted boys])

It is the figurative language that helps Appelfeld to achieve indistinctness and mixes discursive domains as a device for blurring.

Blurring on the Structural Level

Throughout, *Searing Light* generates a network of oppositions in an attempt to illuminate the relations that constitute its main themes. An oppositional pattern consists of opposing concepts, and it is a frequent figure in Appelfeld's novel. Polarity emphasizes contrast and opposition and contributes to an effect of pathos. But a more painstaking look into how the text organizes its materials bears out that the complex use of these forms actually weakens oppositions, undoing their polarity. Pathos as a result is restrained, and themes grow more subtle.[75] Here are some oppositional patterns (not in hierarchical order) that can be traced back to the novel:

a change .... routine
b victim .... aggressor
c adolescents .... adults
d school students .... school staff
e Holocaust survivors .... (pre-)Israeli citizens
f moralists .... nihilists
g memory .... oblivion
h silence ... talk
i health .... sickness/disability
j artists ...tradespeople
k work .... idleness
l sun, light .... darkness, shadow
m individual .... group

These are binary oppositions, divided semantically by a sharp line. These binaries cannot be quantified relatively,[76] and they have an associated value judgment based in social-cultural norms. Sun and light are encoded as positive values, while darkness and shadow are valued negatively. Use of binary opposition issues in dichotomies, which tend to instill expectations of drama and pathos.

This expectation, however, is not fulfilled because Appelfeld uses other devices as well. The result is a tight, saturated, and intensive atmosphere, on the one hand, which remains, on the other, not actualized, reserved, and restrained. The value-laden marking and inversion of the dichotomies blur the nonambivalent distinction between the opposites while also blurring their oppositional tension. This is how the dramatic impression natural to oppositions is attenuated, though never erased. The blurred opposition has the effect of shifting attention from the direct clash between opposites toward the construction of interrelations, which marginalizes the dramatic effect.

One example of how the oppositional structure becomes attenuated is the creation of various evaluative perspectives on the polarity of "change – routine." Throughout the entire novel a demand for constant change is felt. This demand takes on different aspects and acts in two directions. An external demand for a change of character in the boys – this is a didactic-indoctrinating demand coming from the educational institution in which they are enrolled. The other direction takes the form of a demand the boys experience themselves – for personal as well as social change.

Both directions feature change as a positive thing which ought to be pursued and achieved. Toward the end of the novel, a "medical" examination – carried out in the run-up to the boys' conscription – checks the degree of change they have undergone. This is what the text says about Janko: "Janko, though, had changed, he had changed a lot, cast iron in his square shoulders."[77] And this about Shapira: "Shapira changed unrecognizably, right before my eyes. […] Nothing remained of his earlier, boyish appearance" (p. 151). The following words are about Mintz:

> He'd been thin just a few months ago, his trousers loose on his hips, his eyes moist and downcast, hardly ever uttering a syllable. He wasn't even quick. And then, all weaknesses joining together, turned into strength. He straightened up, an evil stubble began to cover his face, and he was all confidence.
>
> (p.64)

The narrator himself is not sure, throughout the novel, which way he should choose. He oscillates between the attempt to hold onto past memories and the attempt to let them go to start a new life. At the end of the novel, he tears up his paintings, which gives him some relief.

The characters' mental changes are reflected in physical ones: "Now you could see how we had grown. Coats were too tight, trousers too short – the sun which had been jabbing at us all through the summer had achieved miracles" (p.149). It appears that within the short period covered by the narrative, the boys experience positive changes. One feels they have managed to break the wall hemming in their lives during the Holocaust and that they are now internalizing the new values pre-state Israel holds out to them. The change pole, perceived as positive, has as its opposite the pole of routine, whose representatives are the tradesmen and the smugglers. They are presented throughout as wholly uninterested in change: they stick to the values they brought with them from overseas. This group is portrayed as a negative group with which the boys as well as the school staff avoid any contact and which they judge harshly. This is illustrated by the encounter between the boys and the tradesmen in Chapter 6. When they meet the tradesmen in café "Rex," the boys, who have already been indoctrinated by Rakush (the dentist), on the one hand, and by school personnel, on the other (the unmarried woman and the janitor), clash with them. In the exchange leading up to this row, the boys identify with the workers' movement, those who are productive, who construct and innovate, while the tradespeople are presented as decadent parasites:

> 'Who are you?', asked one of the traders.
> Mintz answered: 'Farmers.'
> 'One wouldn't say,' said the trader.
> 'Not traders, anyhow.'
> 'What's bad about trade?' wondered the trader
> 'It makes the muscles go weak,' Mintz jested.
>
> (p.50)

Later, during another encounter between the boys, the janitor, and the tradespeople, as they search for Bloch, it is revealed how the more experienced, veteran locals regard the tradesmen:

> The janitor cursed the tradespeople and the smugglers who came only to lay waste to the land with their filthy business. In earlier times, people no sooner arrived or they'd go out to work. Now, after the Holocaust, no one cared for our mission – it was all about merchandise, all about money, and that's how they were defiling what was most precious to us, the very apple of our eye.
>
> (p.110)

The guards have a similar opinion: "The guards would gnash their teeth. We have to do the guarding, and they're idle. Who brought them here. Who needs them. They're messing up the beach" (p.144).

Yet despite this dichotomizing presentation, in which the boys' change-oriented actions are presented as positive and the tradesmen's refusal to change is made out to be negative, elsewhere in the novel this impression turns upside down. All the changes the boys undergo turn out to be irrelevant. That change has happened on a certain level, at some level of intensity or another, to various people, and does not amount to anything much at the novel's ending:

> The truck arrived late at night. The driver, coming out of the cabin, called out angrily: 'Where are they? Where?' [...] The driver pulled the stubborn hook and the door slammed. As in sleep, no need for words. One after the other, the bodies poured into the cargo bed.
>
> (p.155)

The attempts to change are erased at one blow, and the conclusion returns the boys to their anonymous-meaningless origin, the hard, traumatic core which is impenetrable to change.

The tradespeople, in parallel and by contrast, who represent the pole of non-change, sometimes appear to be very stable. Their unchangingness, rather than being presented as an anachronism, appears to mainly suggest consistency and authenticity. For the narrator, consistency offers an anchor in a world ruled by chaos: "I look around: Everything is strange, stranger than on the ship from which we were disgorged tonight" (p.29). Seen as corrupt by the pioneering Zionist community in Eretz Israel, the tradesmen, from the narrator's perspective, appear as warm, delicate, and sensitive people:

> How wonderful they are, the traders, I am suddenly gripped by admiration. If it wasn't for them, their cool, people would be devoured by their madnesses. They – all they've got is their cards changing hands lightly [...] and even though they lack any sincerity, to me they appear warmhearted people.
>
> (pp.31–32)

During the meeting between the janitor and the traders, when they are looking for Blum, one of the latter says something that illustrates the narrator's feelings about them:

> Then one of the tradespeople stepped forward and spoke. He told us calmly how some months ago, the boy Blum came to the shack. [...] So, what were we to do. Throw him out. [...] We too had children once. We would not harm children.
>
> (p.112)

Appelfeld uses the neutralization of opposites as a force holding back feelings that threaten to erupt. Blurring results in a fragmented image, scattering thematic foci in a way that subdues their emotional charge and makes them blend in. The blurring of domains diminishes the salience of charged and raw subject matter and thereby contributes to restraint and reserve.

The Device of Fragmentation

While the device of reduction reduces or leaves out certain details from the text, and blurring helps to blunt details, fragmentation is a device that disconnects between details in the text. This device does not highlight information gaps as much as the cuts and lack of flow caused by these gaps.

Fragmentation on the Level of Syntax

As mentioned, Appelfeld's sentences are delivered staccato-like, in fragments, as though a void lurks right beneath them. The novel is sparse on conjunctions, and the most frequent form of linking between sentences is achieved through additive conjunction, rather than causality. Here is an example:

> February was cold, blue and odorless.
> A chill vapor rose from the wet sand in the afternoons.
> When the haze lifted it exposed a wide and desolate horizon.
> The craving for hot food had not grown less even now, months after the war.
> It was more nagging, biting, now.
> No one knew what else the days would bring.
> The low dunes dragged us from one place to the next.
> This drifting was meaningless – only to keep away from the refugees.
>
> (p.7)[78]

The sense of fragmentation in this passage is the result of an accumulation of syntactic and thematic subjects which remain causally unrelated and fail to add up to a narrative sequence. The quantity of topics and the brevity of the sentences reinforce the autonomy of the parts at the expense of the whole. The resulting image is a pile of details that does not directly and explicitly respond to or is subordinate to a generally coherent framework. Fragmentation, on the level of both the sentence and of the individual words, draws attention away from meaning and toward sound, tone, and rhythm. The novel includes many passages whose musicality dominates and immerses the reader in unconscious contents, remembered bits, and yearning for a lost world. The following lines illustrate this:

> Now I have no one.
> Everything is foreign.
> The few words which I kept throughout the war sigh inside me, ashamed.
> I keep hearing Arthur's thundering.
> No fall left. No birds.
> Only soot.
> You haven't seen any soot.
> Where were you during the war.
>
> (p.60)[79]

Fragmentation on the level of syntax envelops the words with a belt of silence, thereby suggesting something unexpressed yet present.

Fragmentation between a Cluster of Details and Their Generalization

Fragmentation, on the level of language, occurs between the details of description and where they are cut off from their unification under a generalized title. At this cut-off point the cluster of detail may remain without an organizing frame, as we can see here: "he clung to the pods again" (p.73), and alternatively it may issue in a random generalization whose details are missing: "thirst was followed by thirst" (p.128).

Fragmentation between Detail and Whole

Fragmentation also graphically allies itself with the novel's synecdoche. Where fragmentation is achieved by means of synecdoche, the parts of the whole become autonomous, creating an impression of the parts overtaking the whole. A case in point is where fragmentation of the body's parts comes to dominate the whole, which is the embodied "self." This disruption between the body's parts and the whole body serves the sense of fragmentation or crumbling of the "self," together with the insertion of a mechanistic, automatic, not fully conscious dimension into people's action. Here are some illustrations:

> In the long corridor … faces pass in a hurried blur.
>
> (Chapter 7)

> Mouths have learned to mock, smoke, spill out words, and feet to stamp to the beat of the music.
>
> (Chapter 13)

The autonomy of the parts of the whole body and the text's treatment of them as stand-alone entities, helps create a mechanic, soulless mood. The focus of attention is no longer the human being, with their thoughts and feelings, but mechanically operating matter. The mechanization that overtakes the description of parts of reality highlights the neutral, unconscious quality, the automaticity, of life in the shadow of trauma. It is by dissociating from consciousness that existence becomes possible.

Fragmentation on the Structural Level

Searing Light includes seventeen chapters. Each chapter is an entity in its own right describing an experience at a specific place and point in time:

> Chapters 1–2: Description of the boys wandering along the southern Italian coast, during the fall and winter following the end of World War 2. The chapter ends with the boys being taken to the transit camp from which they will immigrate to pre-state Israel.
> Chapter 3: Sailing from Italy to mandatory Palestine. This occurs during the springtime.
> Chapter 4: Description of a day and a night in the transit camp in Palestine.
> Chapters 5–7: The boy's daily life in a residential school, somewhere in the center of the country, near Jaffa. The events occur in the spring, in April.
> Chapters 8–13: The boys' life at residential school during the summer.
> Chapters 14–16: The boys' and school staff's lives during the fall.
> Chapter 17: Description of the boys' military enlistment and training at the end of the summer.

The novel, as can be seen from the above, observes a chronology that follows a naturalistic progression through time. The novel's plot advances by sticking to the temporal sequence of the seasons, from fall to fall. The changes of season are marked by landscape images appropriate to the specific season. The focus is on weather changes: wind and rain in descriptions of winter, heat and light for spring and summer. A positive attitude is markedly absent in these descriptions of time, like references to the renewal of nature in the spring, the appearance of animals, or other aspects of the changing seasons. Nor does the novel mention any of the cultural events associated with the seasons, like Jewish festivals, for instance the celebration of the New Year, the Day of Atonement, the Feast of Huts – all of them related to the fall. The news or historical events are completely absent, even though the narrative occurs just before the outbreak of the independence war.

As a result of this absence of cultural time the characters remain exposed, desolate, to the physical time of the seasons. The chronological frame serves as the glue ensuring minimal narrative coherence. Without that formal frame the materials will stand revealed in their isolation, cut off from any meaning-bearing form.

The novel's fragmented details illuminate the fragmented and broken nature of reality. Fragmentation and dissociation lead to discontinuity, disruption, and weakens what can be considered "good" form. When form becomes loose it weakens – allowing for emotional intensities, which will not be registered consciously, to become submerged.

The Device of Equivalence

This device operates by attributing equal importance to all of the text's materials. This can be achieved by canceling two elements crucial to constructing a coherent whole: the text's causal structure, and its hierarchical structure.

Canceling the Causal Structure

Aristotle in his *Poetics* argued that a text will be unified wherever there is a causal relation between its events, such that each event can be understood in terms of the one preceding it, or leads of necessity or logically to the one following it. The parts will be structurally linked in such a manner that if and when one part is displaced or removed, the whole will collapse: wherever the presence or absence of a part is unnoticeable, it is not an organic part of the whole.[80] Even though *Searing Light* creates an impression of wholeness, due to its chronological, apparently realistic, sequence, it does not meet Aristotle's criterion of unity. The novel's chronological order actually only gives it an appearance of unity, as its chapters are stand-alone units whose order is interchangeable, or can even be published in its own right. Thus indeed, the novel's Chapter 3 was published separately, as a chapter entitled "1946" in another one of Appelfeld's books *Essays in the First Person*.[81]

Appelfeld seems to have consciously given up on the principle of causality, and replaced it by another principle, that of analogy. He adopts a narrative principle that rather than following a horizontal, causal movement, follows a vertical, analogous one which emerges as the result of an equivalence between the chapters.[82]

Canceling the Hierarchical Structure

Appelfeld's novel does not observe the classic hierarchic structure. This is because rather than having one main center, the novel presents us with several centers which are equivalent in terms of importance. Arnheim defines the center of a work of art as follows: "[...] the center of a field of forces, a focus from which forces issue and toward which forces converge."[83]

Though *Searing Light* has no obvious center of gravity, such a center can nevertheless be traced through its remaining small foci. This disintegration at the novel's core affects its structure. A macro-textual observation at the manner in which the novel's chapters are linked reveals an interesting phenomenon. The novel would seem to follow the traditional dramatic scheme: exposition, complication, crisis, resolution, coda. Here, the exposition covers the first chapters,

1–4, which are dedicated to a description of the boys, Holocaust survivors, who are now in Italy and making their way to mandatory Palestine. The entanglement or complication stage (Chapters 5–13) consists of the boys' difficulties at arrival, their adjustment, and their attempt to become part of life in their new country. It would seem that resolution is reached (Chapters 15 and 16) with the description of the staff at the residential school; this is also the point in the narrative when they themselves are told about the fate of their families in the Holocaust. The coda takes the shape of the novel's final chapter (17), which narrates the boys' enlistment to the army, constituting a kind of conclusion to the entire sequence of events.

If we follow the classic order, Chapter 14, which I did not mention above, should take the role of the novel's turning point – that is to say: its center of gravity – and it is placed between the part describing the children who are now being educated at the institution, and the one describing the institution's workers. In fact, this chapter does present emotional material, supporting the idea that it forms the novel's peak. Here is where the protagonist comes face to face with himself and grows conscious of his most deeply hidden shame: his having been abandoned by his father when the war broke out:

> The war put an end to many of our feelings but not my little disgrace. At night in the half-light of sleep I feel it strongly. Every so often I ask, once again, whether my father intended to abandon us or was it a moment's whim.
>
> (p.116)

Here the chapter exposes the protagonist's vulnerability even in the world that preceded the Holocaust. Appelfeld generalizes the disintegration associated with the Holocaust to human existence as a whole, with the Holocaust featuring as an especially powerful eruption of profound, ongoing principle.

If we refer to Arnheim's above definition in relation to Appelfeld's novel, we can think of Chapter 14 as the center around which its subject matter arranges itself. Indeed, while the chapters leading up to it are devoted to the boys' apprehensions and their ways of coping (or their failure to cope) with the physical as well as mental desolation following their families' extermination, the chapters following it, all the way to the novel's end, look at the school staff's engagement with the same pain, the same fate.

The novel's move to a description of these employees' vulnerability – people who until then have appeared heartless, insensitive, as if they had never suffered themselves – expands the circle of victims, and undoes the dichotomy resulting from the conflict between pupils and staff. With the description of Clara's madness, and the janitor's quiet depression, we now have a human document including all of the novel's figures.

Chapter 14 is located between the two opposing extremes: the boys and the school staff. So that in terms of both its structural position and its contents, this chapter can be expected to be the most emotionally charged.

Assuming that our examination of the devices Appelfeld uses in order to create an effect of restraint should devote special attention to the text's emotionally most charged spot – the center of gravity to which its dramatic and pathetic forces are directed and from which they derive – we should have a look how the device of equivalence operates here. A micro-textual consideration of the text shows that this chapter, which according to the conventional narrative scheme should be the one in which the story culminates, its center, falls apart into a series of stories and stories within stories, a succession of episodes. The chapter splits apart into two main stories that unfold in different places and times: the story about the boys' stroll through Jaffa, and that about the talk given by the school's unmarried woman. And each of these splits up into further, secondary stories, resulting in a central chapter consisting of a number of expanded centers. The unified form crumbles, with the input shifting from one pivot to another, as if in an attempt to find an organizing principle that might restore unity to the narrative bits and pieces.

Arnheim, in his analysis of Mondrian,[84] also argued that if the text is disintegrated and scattered, it loses its hierarchical structure to a homogenous one where importance is equally distributed. Taking this into account, the splitting of the plot in Chapter 14 is not by coincidence, and it joins the final Chapter 17 which concludes with an open ending, in creating the conditions for converting the sequentially evolving dramatic structure into an alternative structure based in equivalence. As the novel's center is fragmented, the search for another center which will organize the entire story hierarchically, proves to be fruitless. Instead of a main, central junction, local centers pop up and the only connectivity between them that could possibly yield a meaningful structure is a connectivity based in equivalence. This connectivity has the effect of eliminating priorities: nothing appears as more or less important than anything else. This device takes direct and sharp attention from the emotionally charged materials and scatters it equally among all the novel's materials.

The Open Ending

The novel's final chapter describes the boys' joining the army. This situation which more than anything else might have signaled their possible release from trauma's fate, actually takes the boys back to where they started, a return to the set model of the past: they move on to yet another camp. The novel, in this sense, concludes with an endless repetition of the traumatic past: life in camps.

This return of the "closed camp"[85] in the novel's final episode – "Appelfeld's penal colony," as Schwartz called it[86] – produces a clash between the infinitely open structure, content-wise, and the novel's formally closed structure. This clash results in an illusory sense of the final episode somehow breaking through the novel's natural boundaries, continuing to resonate beyond its concluding outline. This is how the sense of infinity, which Arnheim mentions in his analysis of Mondrian's painting, comes into being.[87] An unresolved sense of infinity is one feature of the open ending,[88] an ending which also participates in the conversion of the hierarchical structure into a homogenous one that tends to infinity.

The hierarchical structure's conversion into a homogenous one is supported on the novel's thematic level, where Appelfeld depicts a meaningless world: "No one knew what else the future would bring. The low sands drove us this way and that. This drifting was wholly meaningless" (p.7). This drifting from one place to another and along the axis of time forms the novel's pivot. In this sense, each chapter is a reflection of the inability to cope with the meaning of the world in the wake of the Holocaust.

Yet at the end of the novel, traditional elements are brought to achieve, to some extent, a closure. So, for instance, many of the figures who have appeared in the course of the novel, now, at its end, come together on the occasion of the boys' enlistment, which is treated as a concluding event. The description of a human experience issues in departure, moving out into an unknown future, as well as the compositional choice of season and time – the end of summer and of the day – may all contribute to a sense of a proper conclusion.[89] All of these traditional elements prevent the disintegration of an open ending and allow the theme to rein in chaos.

Avoiding Conceptualization – Discourse on Low-Level of Organization

All these above devices – reduction, blurring, fragmentation, and equivalence – create a form of expression that seeks to present the traumatic experience at a low level of organization. Appelfeld employs primary, basic and distinct forms of the kind that children will find easily accessible, while interfering with them through deformations that come to weaken and undo them. In so doing, Appelfeld succeeds in creating a pre-symbolic mode of expression for representing traumatic experience. He uses powerful, basic forms exactly because their disintegration offers him a way into unconscious materials that have neither been generalized nor abstracted. I believe that his success at getting through to these pre-symbolic "zones" is path breaking where it comes to the symbolic representation of traumatic reality. The following examples illustrate the choice of basic forms and their disintegration by means of these devices:

In the Domain of Language: Appelfeld uses deixis in relation to the spatio-temporal frame of his novel, yet he leaves it void of the object to which expression was supposed to refer. I called this linguistic phenomenon a hollow deixis which causes a regression to the pre-symbolic domain.

In the Domain of Figurative Language: Appelfeld has a predilection for sensory metaphors, in which, due to a shared sensory feature, object A is perceived as object B (shape and color; movement and sound). Conceptually based, abstract metaphors appear infrequently. This is also related to the choice of a simple and basic level of organization. Research has shown that children prefer metaphor over literal expression, only when the metaphor's comparative basis is sensory: at earlier stages of development, form and color; next, sound and movement. Conceptually based metaphor becomes the preferred mode at an older age.[90] Where Appelfeld uses sensory metaphors whose comparative basis is shape, texture, or color – texture and color are more prominent than those that refer to shape: "The nights were falling warm and dark as if made of black fluff" (p.63). Reference to colors without concrete shape, and a texture whose outline is indistinct allows him to go beyond the obvious and apparent. This leads to a special, paradoxical quality of concreteness. An intangible, undefined concreteness.

In the Structural Domain: Appelfeld deploys dichotomous as well as paratactic structures. Dichotomy is considered a basic, primary mode of thinking. Appelfeld uses it as the minimal entity representing extremes and oppositions. Dichotomy creates order among elements by opposing them to each other. And yet, I have shown how the validity of dichotomy comes under question in Appelfeld's writing when he relates inconsistently to opposing poles. This is how the strong form weakens and disintegrates, not just on the level of language, but structurally as well.

A paratactic structure is a disintegrated hierarchical structure. With the undoing of its pivotal center, the novel *Searing Light* becomes a sequence of chapters that connect on a basis of equivalence. Herrnstein-Smith observes that paratactic structures can often be found in children's poetry, lullabies, or folk-songs.[91] So here too, Appelfeld can be seen to use primary forms that are simple and clear but only to weaken and undo them at a later stage. He achieves this by undermining his novel's center of gravity, as I have illustrated in analyzing Chapter 14, as well as by interfering with the narrative's closure. The open ending gets in the way of the paratactic structure eventually becoming solid and stable, so that the book remains at a low level of organization in narrative terms as well.

To conclude: This part of my examination has looked at the poetic defense mechanisms available to a restrained style. Appelfeld used language materials that construct basic, extremely clear forms, then took them apart, in order thus to attain a pre-symbolic level of writing which, in his view, is the most appropriate form of expression in regard of trauma. Material in a pre-symbolic state renders an intensive and saturated mood and vague atmosphere; it does not allow for distinct definition. This is how Appelfeld achieves the saturated mood that enables him to touch upon the emotionally charged material yet not to conceptualize it.

Jointly these devices – reduction, blurring, fragmentation, and equivalence – produce a singular poetic expression that results in a highly blunted text. While managing to achieve a saturated atmosphere, he avoids to directly conceptualize the charged material. He does not remove or neutralize this charged feeling; he guides his reader to it only to apply, when the time is ripe, the above devices which conceal it. This issue is a tense constellation which causes the reader an intense experience, reaching the very cusp of conceptualization, then to be left with an unfocused feeling which declines any form of categorization.[92] These poetic devices constitute the textual defense system which helps us consider the author's mental coping strategies with catastrophic experience.

Appelfeld's use of mechanisms of restraint in *Searing Light*, I have shown, served the need to represent the traumatic memory on a pre-symbolic level, memory experienced through sensations and feelings, rather than cognition. I believe that these mechanisms are traces of a psychic formation, part of which includes coping via acting-out, and another processing.

Pre-symbolic representation, I argue, is a type of memory inscription that occurs in especially dire situations. This type of memory attempts to present suppressed experiences by means of merely iconic, sensory language.[93] The presence of a traumatic memory, then, is felt intensively and densely, yet cannot be felt as a symbolically identifiable experience. Mediated to the reader through language, this memory is experienced on the most fundamental level of existence, that of the body. It is body memory, not mental memory, that preserves most trenchantly the terror, rage, and pain of the traumatic experience of loss.[94]

The Poetics of Body Memory

Post-traumatic stress disorder (PTSD) has been defined, among other things, as a disease of time,[95] with the past infiltrating and activating the traumatic memory in the present. Restoring time's chronological order by creating a narrative, is one therapeutic means to achieve release from trauma and the restructuring of the disintegrated personality. For Appelfeld, however, putting time into chronological order may interfere with his ability to express experience authentically. Memoir writing tends to wrap the burning interior in many external facts in an attempt for it never to be exposed – and this is not what he, as an artist, seeks. Appelfeld's writing is definitely not what he calls memoir writing:

> What I am trying to do is not to write a present, but to bring up from inside my lost time, and to see what might be its meaning in relation to "general", ongoing time. I therefore am neither dealing with the present, nor with memoir-writing [...] Initially I wrote stories whose autobiographical element was easily recognizable, but later I put them away, with the same wish to bring my inner time into contact with the flow of the present.[96]

Many published testimonies about the Holocaust are, for Appelfeld, repressions "whose only function is to put time into chronological order."[97] Among this wealth of accounts, "which only grew over time, the inner voice of the 'self' was in hiding, locked away behind seven bars."[98] This is the voice Appelfeld tried to release and render audible. In another interview he said:

> My work is memorial, yet it is an absent memory. I was seven years old when the war broke out. I make a reconstruction which begins in total blindness... At the deep origin of things there is a seed of memory... I was too young to bring things to consciousness.[99]

Appelfeld admits he has no access to this memory.

> I don't remember even one of the villages all across Ukraine I passed through in fear. I was in the company of hundreds of refugees and I remember not even one name. The war crushed you. Everything became one long dark convoy to the unknown.[100]

And yet this memory is alive, more than any other factual recollection. This type of memory gets imprinted in the flesh and is felt on the bodily level, and in this sense, it is the most authentic memory.[101] Appelfeld's terror was inscribed in his body and became one with it.[102] In another interview he said:

> Children have no chronology… A very famous poet, Paul Celan, said that the war was like black milk… it's part of your organism, not in the sense that you have any control or power over it, but that it becomes part of your cells.[103]

Rather than the reflective perspective, conscious of itself, it is the vibrant contact with authentic material that body memory renders:

> You see, my childhood unfolded under unnatural circumstances. I spent much time in camps, fields, orchards, forests, in the homes of Christians. So that what I mainly learned was touch. They didn't teach me intellect.[104]

Schwartz argues[105] that recollection in Appelfeld is "artificial": knowledge acquired and processed at a later stage is presented as the author's basic experience. This raises a question about the nature of recollection: Does it consist of a type of presenting sensations without cognition's involvement, in an attempt to create/represent body memory by means of poetic language, or is it based on subsequently acquired knowledge, as Schwartz suggests? Is it a process of anamnesis, as in Lyotard's view,[106] in which the unknown is allowed to emerge, the unseen to show through, or is it a semantic processing of a memory produced from external information? What, in Appelfeld's process of recollection, passes through the poetic device of restraint – a process of inner impoverishment aimed to help represent the traumatic core – and what, by contrast, is the result of a process of artificial construction consisting of external knowledge, as Schwartz would have it.

Discussing Appelfeld's "imaginary autobiography" in the novella "The Age of Wonder,"[107] Schwartz argues that most of the novella's details were collected from Appelfeld's knowledge about Jewish history in the past century in general, and more specifically that of the assimilated Jewish community of Bukovina in the inter-war years. He considers "The Age of Wonder" a fragmented, imaginary autobiographical novella, whose design reflects a lack of distinction between biographical reality, on the one hand, and dream or nightmare, on the other.[108]

I believe that Appelfeld uses actual and fictional childhood recollections alike as condensed emotional material to help him reach the concealed memory of trauma. This is literary fiction – not academic, historical writing, and Appelfeld uses body memory as the dimension that allows him to approach the traumatic core as closely as possible, the secret, death, to touch yet not quite touch it. This is Appelfeld's non-memoir, his poetic testimony. He rejects the language of memoir writing, commenting that to him it is an envelope consisting of many external facts, one externalization after another to ensure that what's inside will never see the light of day.[109]

It is the sense of loss and absence about his past that is the moving force and main impulse behind Appelfeld's work. His way of coping with this past is a long process of recollection (anamnesis) with memory time and again being made present through acting-out. These materials are filtered and processed by means of the textual defense mechanisms. Appelfeld compared himself to an architect:

> ...not of one house but of an entire neighborhood. In my head I carry the image of the whole neighborhood. I know exactly where the trees are, where a house is missing...Can you imagine how many years I will have to live in order to complete the whole neighborhood?[110]

Like Scheherazade in *One Thousand and One Nights*, Appelfeld gains meaningful existence through the daily drawing and construction of the "neighborhood" stories he extracts from oblivion. His task is to bring the past into an eternal present which will always be present.[111]

Appelfeld's mental struggle in *Searing Light* does not lead to a redemptive solution. It seems to me that Appelfeld never undoes the Gordian knot between himself and his past. The past dwells with him like a forever open wound. His childhood uprooting and orphanhood, together with the sense of terrible loss, are his guiding, ongoing experience, and over the course of time these became the crux of his work. He has a constant need to revisit his traumatic childhood which has become inscribed in his body, in order to try and salvage, from this abyss, the real memories. The world of the past includes the deprivation of his uprooted childhood, yet is also responsible for the desire and yearning to fill this void. This is the inner world that enables him to envision a unified space, in which he can revert to his lost parents and merge with them and look for redemption from his orphanhood. This desire is powerfully felt toward the end of the novel *All Whom I Have Loved*,[112] as well as at the end of this novel.[113] The fact that the protagonist is left with the same profound yearning for symbiosis, and with the refusal to recognize that this wish can never be realized, refers to an existential condition that profoundly and touchingly represents the experience of deprivation, of trauma. Giving voice to the self that went into hiding and silence during the years of the war is the processing Appelfeld finds in art: "I know by now that it cannot be fully understood, and [in my writing] I am moving, rather, in the direction of someone who tried to grasp something encountered in the past which he keeps examining, each time anew."[114] While psychologically speaking it is impossible to escape trauma, art turns into a safe space from which Appelfeld observes trauma, something which he can contain through writing.

This search for the authentic core of experience and the personal voice to express it, doesn't absolve Appelfeld from the need to find the proper distance to look at things. He believes that aesthetic distance is a condition for good art. This distance requires to move away from a memoirist approach to experience, from historical chronology, and from using the act of writing as a form of therapy. He explains how he was already beyond therapy by the time he came to write: "Writing is a stage of consciousness that goes beyond therapy. It is not a good thing for writing to be involved in a therapeutic process. One must dwell in a certain distance in order to write."[115]

Appelfeld's distancing is for the sake of an authentic return to, and contact with the source by means of his singular poetic language.

Appelfeld, as I already wrote, said that people tend to envelope the great catastrophes with words that seek to protect themselves. He, by contrast, tried to go back and touch the wordlessness that took hold of him following trauma.[116] His great question is: How does one put this burning matter into words? How to touch this resounding dusk? How to approach this muted domain of silence with language?

In *Searing Light*, writing as an activity does not yet feature. Instead, the language of the body, as Kristeva called it,[117] emerges through Appelfeld's poetic writing. It is only at a later stage in Appelfeld's oeuvre, in the novel *The Man Who Never Stopped Sleeping*, that writing itself becomes present.[118] Discussing the language of poetry, Kristeva seeks to bring back the language of the body to the human sciences.[119] Body language, she believes, is in the domain of poetic language. Kristeva is interested in the limits of language: the places where it is constituted (through the processes of language acquisition) and those where it disintegrates (through psychotic fragmentation). She distinguishes between semiotic and symbolic elements. The semiotic consists of the operationalization of the drives, which in language takes the form of sound, rhythm and tune. They mark the physical basis of language, beyond the semiotic language stops to exist as such.[120] The symbolic is the structure or grammar that controls how meaning comes about. For Kristeva, the semiotic is the component of meaning that is related to the drives and emotions. The semiotic, in other words, is the corporeal element of language, while the symbolic is the ideational component.

Poetic language, according to Kristeva, operates in the domain between what she calls the genotext and the phenotext. The genotext is the driving force underlying language, while the phenotext is the structural, grammatical force which makes communication possible. The distinction between genotext and phenotext corresponds with that between semiotic and symbolic. Poetic language, Kristeva believes, has the capacity to resurrect language's instinctual forces through sound and rhythm.

In her analysis, Kristeva looks back to Lacan's formative concepts of the real, the imaginary and the symbolic. The real is the domain of lack; the imaginary is the domain of signifiers, and the symbolic is the domain which bestows linguistic value on signifiers.[121] Lack constantly troubles and shocks the psyche. In Kristeva's view,[122] poetic language carries the traces of lack, and its role is to unsettle the symbolic order, to expose the crack and make lack present and visible. Kristeva regards the real as the authentic, and the semiotic approaches it most closely, while the symbolic is remote and more deceptive. Poetic language breaks the order of the symbolic and takes us, still within the domain of language, closer, via the semiotic, to the real, and to lack.

Even so, Kristeva also argues that poetic language does not entirely forfeit the symbolic: it only disrupts it by means of the semiotic. The semiotic system cannot substitute for the symbolic order, it doesn't constitute a language we can use instead of normal discourse. While a psychotic state should not completely crush the symbolic order, the latter should not stunt expression, without access to the real. It is poetic language that makes the encounter between the real and the symbolic possible without taking the path of madness or fabrication. She introduces a dynamic within the conventional system of signification by questioning its limits.

Kristeva seeks to clarify how absence – the unconscious, the inexpressible – is rendered in language. She examines the unconscious from the perspective of poetic language, the semiotic, expression through sound, music and rhythm. Language's concreteness points at the semiotic body that at one and same time constitutes as well as undoes language.[123] Referring to Kristeva, I here suggest three distinctive features – music, stutter, and the intangible concrete – which in the case of Appelfeld's poetic language preserve the memory of the body, which is responsible for the elusive contact he makes with the traumatic core.

The Musical Element

"I understood that realism could not always serve my purpose," said Appelfeld in another interview,

> One method I employed was language as a musical tool. I have not always used words from their content-related aspect. I went for the music, the vibration – not just of a word, but of a sentence or passage. I invest some effort into shaping a passage into a melody.[124]

The memory of the lost home, on the one hand, and the terrifying forests that were his hiding place during the war, on the other, animated, he said, the Hebrew characters with a powerful and rhythmic melody which never since left him.[125]

The Element of Stutter

Stutter constitutes the representation of body memory in language. Appelfeld is not a great believer in words. Words, for him come to cover up trauma.[126] The loss of the few words he actually had to his disposal comes to serve him by offering authentic and sincere access to the unknown world he confronts:

> I am not a great admirer of the fluent word, I am more of a believer in stutter. We might be organized when things flow, but stutter allows for the friction between feeling and thought, and that's what I'm interested in. I want my protagonists to discover themselves, their inner lives. That is why they find themselves frustrated – with the inability to express themselves. This muteness is immanent, in some sense. The protagonists in my books don't suffer from some intellectual or emotional defect, my protagonists know that they don't know […] words are limited because our ability to think is limited, and because our feelings are not always clear.[127]

Here Appelfeld indicates the need to find the form that will most faithfully represent language's insufficiency where it encounters trauma of this proportion. Two of his novels *All Whom I Have Loved,*[128] and *The Journey into Winter,*[129] illustrate the tension between speech and silence, and the stutter in between them. As early as in his *Essays in the First Person*, where he discusses the language of Y.H. Brenner, Appelfeld says that the one who searches for his truth speaks in a profound stutter, out of a seething, abominable frustration, reachng out for a savior which cannot be found whether within or without. This seems to reflect Appelfeld's own search for the right words, and in this search stuttering comes to his assistance.[130]

The Element of Intangible Concreteness

Appelfeld's style grew more lucid over the years.[131] His writing increasingly shed all unnecessary ornamentation, and the language grew more concrete, devoid of symbolism or allegory. Appelfeld sought simple and literal expression. The figures' physical existence came first:

> I look at people from my personal perspective. I look at facial expressions, the movements of their hands, shoulders, the nose, and this too is how I write. The physis comes before anything. Once you capture the physis, the psyche follows.[132]

For Appelfeld body movement is more truthful than thought. "When I look at a person, more than listening to his thoughts and trying to judge them, I examine the movements of his body, his face, arms, legs, his posture. I believe that is much more informative."[133] Still concreteness à la Appelfeld, as I explained with reference to *Searing Light*, is of a special kind which I would venture to call an *intangible concreteness*. It is this intensive, condensed feeling he creates, originating in the body, concrete, but because its outlines are removed it turns intangible, leaving us with a powerfully compressed sensation.

Rachel Albeck-Gidron argues that Appelfeld's literary forms of grief are unique in literature, appearing as a type of loss a kind of a lexical loss, a loss of the sign itself.[134] I ask: Do the traces of absence already constitute a sign? Doesn't this sign, of the last one contrive to point at absence in the most present, concrete of ways? A sign that echoes the condensed nature of the experience of loss. Making the traces of absence present, even if only by way of an empty reality, intangible yet condensed, and marked by its boundaries – this is what constitutes Appelfeld's desperate struggle to validate the reality of trauma and to fight the inability to represent it. Loss is not a sign but a thing whose presence can be validated even in its absence.

Appelfeld's poetic language, with its melody, stutter, and its intangible concreteness, enables the return into language of the repressed, while the mechanisms of reduction I presented help the absent to manifest itself in language in a controlled manner, avoiding madness, or worse: falsity. These three features help present experience in the very most primary form language can attain as it approaches the authentic core of trauma. This representation is achieved through the processing and development of Appelfeld's unique poetic diction.

We may say, then, that Appelfeld's Holocaust experience goes on living inside him as a present-and-absent acting-out from which no release is to be found. Within the domain of poetic writing, however, he does attain some form of processing, of working through, a form of coping that does not give up lingering and making contact with the traumatic core, while opting to do this from the protected space of poetic language. Appelfeld expresses things that straddle the boundary between language and wordlessness. He penetrates the abyss but does not surrender language's organized and balanced dimension: "For me, writing is a combination of darkness and reason."[135]

The Religious Sublime

In the first section of this chapter, we saw how Appelfeld's restrained style or moderation subserves the textual defense mechanisms used in *Searing Light*, and how these enable him to look into chaos. In the second section, these defense mechanisms revealed how the author mentally worked with the memory of trauma: which included the use of acting-out as well as of working through. Extreme trauma leaves its impact on the child's psyche which subsequently is in thrall to it. Nevertheless, writing poetically about the experience did restore the sense of lost self to Appelfeld, even a feeling that God made man in his image. In this final section, I will make the connection between the Holocaust experience, including the associated acting-out and working through, and a liberating religious experience taking Appelfeld's speaker into new domains, which can be gleaned from the novel *The Man Who Never Stopped Sleeping*.[136]

The experience of the unspeakable excess reminds of a paradigm in the field of aesthetics, namely the sublime. In theories of art and in philosophy the sublime features as a phenomenon defined by its size and intensity, its extreme impact on the subject, and by the way it is represented in terms of the subject's abilities to contain it. Because I find that there is much in common between written representations of the events of the Holocaust and those of the sublime, some clarification of the latter concept may well cast light on the poetic rhetoric of the Holocaust – and more particularly, the manner in which the author's shock is represented. Because of sublimity's association with the divine the connection with the Holocaust's ultimate evil does not seem immediately apparent. Still, if the source of intensity of ultimate evil involves three variables – the size of its object; the subject's position in relation to the size of this object, and questions regarding modes of representation – we might consider it a negative sublime.[137]

The poetic texts produced by Holocaust survivors which I have examined in this book display an irreparable breach, one of whose expressions is radical disintegration of the self. The self has to testify to an experience that is beyond words, which leaves an inaccessible, inconceivable and non-representable void – a residue that refuses articulation. In the poetic texts of the writers, I am considering we can observe an effort to find release from radical evil by means of an act of reframing. This reframing shifts the survivor-witness away from an experience of extreme distress imposed by a negative sublime to an experience of mental elevation achieved by the ability to connect with the positive sublime, whose hidden sources are beyond the self and have the potential to empower it.

In her *Walking Beyond Trauma*[138] Haviva Pedaya proposes a discussion in terms combining the research on trauma and that on ritual and mourning. She looks at ritual as allowing movement of a kind that is between acting-out and working through. In the same vein I would like to propose a discursivity in which the experience of the negative sublime offers a poetic resource which thus leads the writers to an inverse movement toward release from the traumatic experience and toward an experience of the transcendental sublime. Such a breakthrough seems to support the redemption of the torn psyche. Appelfeld, Ka-Tzetnik, and Primo Levi, each in their own way, all include the sublime in their work. In the case of Appelfeld, I will first discuss the self's distress in the face of the negative sublime, in the face of trauma as it appears in *Searing Light*. Then I will show how three drafts composed prior to the act of writing of the first chapter of the imagined book the hero planned to write in *The Man Who Never Stopped Sleeping* reflect the actual transition from the distress of the negative sublime, of the unexpressed residue, to a breach into revelation embodied in poetic writing.

The Holocaust as Negative Sublime in *Searing Light*

In his books *From Individual Lament to Tribal Eternity*[139] and *The Narrative Art of Aharon Appelfeld*[140] Yigal Schwartz set out to follow Appelfeld's "religious journey." Appelfeld's protagonists' journey, he argues, does not lead through institutional religious Judaism – which, by the author's own admission, is outside his existential-emotional domain.[141] Schwartz points out two alternative paths. One of them leads toward Hasidic Judaism, and the other toward the possible birth of a new religion, a Jewish-Christian-Pagan blend. The latter, for Schwartz, constitutes the deepest expression of Appelfeld's religious position.[142]

Even though he did deal with Jewish identity on the collective level, Appelfeld's own take on Judaism derives from a more personal spot. This is what he said in his *Essays in the First Person*: "We dwell deep within a Jewish intimacy. Not theories – but living people; not places – but warm corners"[143] The concept of religiosity, in Appelfeld's work, is perceived from an emotional-experiential position as a sublime. His style basically agrees with Edmund Burke's[144] and Jean-Francois Lyotard's[145] assumptions about the sublime, which refer on the one hand to the impossibility to understand it due to its proportions, intensity and volume and on the other to the terror it instills on the subject due to the inherent life-threatening violence and horror.

Neither the senses, nor the imagination or reason can comprehend the Holocaust. At its center is a terror which mobilizes all of the individual's powers of being. Both Burke ([1757] 1990) and Lyotard (1993) discussed the question of representation in this context. Burke talked about the various forms of experience that unsettle the possibility to register and illustrate how the senses collapse in the face of the phenomenon, causing the appearance of a sense of terror. Vagueness and lack of clarity play a powerful role in producing terror, and this power is crucial, for Burke, in evoking the effect of the sublime.[146] In my discussion of *Searing Light* I showed that Appelfeld's use of literary devices leads to an impression of vagueness of a pre-conceptual kind, something which has the effect of amplifying mental distress, a state of mind without focus or conceptualization.

In Burke's view it is succession and uniformity that produce the destructive whole and represent its size which is beyond the senses' grasp.[147] The conclusion of Appelfeld's *Searing Light*, which in the context of the device of equivalence is an open ending, repeats itself without resolution. This ending, moreover, locks the novel's characters into a "closed camp model" which in the end turns the fragmentary memories of their lives into a tragic homogenous succession: Every new experience the characters encounter follows the archetypal model of the "camp," i.e., the concentration camp.

In Lyotard's reflections on the sublime a special place is reserved for silence. Silence signals expression's admission of failure. Silence renders the inevitable hiatuses of understanding. Silence suggests something beyond our understanding, the trauma which in spite of being present cannot be articulated. Lyotard mentions the traces of what cannot be represented.[148] He turns to artists asking them to invent suggestions and traces of the negative sublime in order to express human insufficiency. With his language of moderation, closer to silence than to screaming, Appelfeld, more than anything, attempts to make absence present.

The Subject's Religious Experience in the Face of the Negative Sublime: Such is the horror produced in the subject's facing the Holocaust that it threatens to unsettle the very existence of the self.[149] In his essay, *At the Mind's Limits*,[150] Jean Améry mentions the fragmentation of self that follows physical torture. Améry, who joined the anti-Nazi resistance, was arrested and tortured by the Gestapo and put into a concentration camp. He mentions how the boundaries of his body, which were the boundaries of his self, were trampled with the first blow. He experienced this boundary breaking as the annihilation of self.[151]

Appelfeld, unlike Améry, does not refer to the biological self – which, in his view, did everything it could to survive, and into which the hidden information of trauma was deposited – but rather to the self as an inclusive spiritual quality, the very essence of the human spirit. It is, for him, from this site of injury that "religiosity distress"[152] emerges. Appelfeld's religiosity distress is a subjective spiritual state of mind, rather than an institutional one. He underwent the apocalyptic terror of the Holocaust, he said, as a deep religious experience, which originated not far off from nihilism.[153] Even though he was writing about Brenner, it would not be farfetched to say that Appelfeld's felt Brenner's type of religiosity alive in himself. So Appelfeld's religiosity originates in a sense of terror vis a vis traumatic experience. It relates to the most profound distress the subject feels in the face of the negative sublime. Burke speaks about the same distress in facing the sublime when he mentions the void, dark, loneliness and silence expressing the terror of the unforeseen, losing one's way and losing coherence. This distress, he believes, gives rise to the typical sense of awe and hallowedness attending the sublime.[154]

Awe, in the case of Appelfeld, takes on a very personal character. His religious distress originates in a personal, subjective experience,[155] which he renders in the domain of art. It is in its safety that Appelfeld attempts to redeem the self, and to transform it, in the wake of the experience of the Holocaust, into a specific, unique self:

> Though art cannot replace faith, its very existence constantly challenges the human's anonymization. The human being is not merely some unstable molecule in violent historical processes, but rather an entire being which will seek, desperately even, for not just its place but also its redemption.[156]

Appelfeld regards authentic literary writing as redemptive, because it can reclaim the individual facing disintegration in the encounter with the negative sublime[157] His obsessive preoccupation with reclaiming the self from arbitrariness assumes that there is an inaccessible, unconscious deep memory, which from its hiding place threatens identity and requires constant confrontation. Focus on freeing the body memory, the biological-physical memory, turns into a preoccupation with the question of the subject's identity.[158] This is where the search after the self begins. Appelfeld makes contact with trauma by dealing with the question of identity – which he tackles by seeking a primary body memory, a positive memory that skirts trauma. This heroic attempt seeks to join positive, empowering forces, not just those of his own earliest years, but – by means of a journey back, across the generations – the Jewish collective memory reaching back all the way to the times of his protagonist's ancestor, Rabbi Sagi Nahor, in *The Man Who Never Stopped Sleeping*. From this search, Appelfeld the artist and individual extracts the powers that help restore his crumbling identity. I will illustrate this journey with reference to the above novel, *The Man Who Never Stopped Sleeping*.[159]

From Excess to Origin: *The Man Who Never Stopped Sleeping*

Here, I would like to draw a link between trauma, religiosity and the art of writing by means of a journey toward the origin. The path of this particular journey attempts to circumvent the traumatic experience by aiming for a place and time prior to it, from which it might be possible to forge and construct a new world. Access to this primordial vanishing point is not possible without passing through the experience of religious elevation which lifts up the broken subject and may release him from his helplessness.[160] The fictional world of poetic writing is the site where this transcendent journey in time is made possible. I will elucidate this through an analysis of the novel *The Man Who Never Stopped Sleeping*.

The novel follows the boy Irwin's long journey, starting with the end of the Second World War in Europe, and continuing to pre-state Israel on the eve of the independence war. Called "the sleeping boy" by the other refugees, the boy is in an ongoing state of slumber, which is periodically interrupted by stretches of wakefulness. The other Holocaust refugees with whom he travels, carry him on their shoulders until they reach the Italian coast. When he arrives to Palestine, he joins the Zionist paramilitary Haganah youth division. On his first military mission he is injured in both his legs, he is hospitalized and undergoes lengthy treatment. Both during his time in hospital, and later in the recovery home, a search unfolds after both his personal identity and his vocation as a writer. Irwin tries to write a book. At the end of *The Man Who Never Stopped Sleeping* he reaches the final draft of the first chapter of his novel, his "first home," where he tries, as he puts it, to drink water from the well of life. As a novel about a novel, *The Man Who Never Stopped Sleeping* is a work of meta-fiction dealing especially with the early stages of writing.

Irwin, in *The Man Who Never Stopped Sleeping*, copes with trauma by writing. He makes failed attempts to achieve a final draft of the first chapter for his yet unwritten book. I will follow these attempts until Irwin completes the first chapter. I will show how these drafts constitute a paradigm for a narrative that circumvents a state of traumatic distress; a narrative that proceeds through a religious experience toward the sanctification of the hero as a writer.

Appelfeld criticism, argues Schwartz, suffers a blind spot due to its obsessive clinging to what he calls the "trauma-sublimation model."[161] On this model a traumatic experience undergoes poetic repetition which allows control and regulation. Schwartz claims that in his later work, Appelfeld attempts to insert into the literary sound box, phantom voices by means of which he may be in touch with the world of the dead. For Schwartz, these voices signal a shift in Appelfeld's work which moved from the personal, psychological to a broader perspective with a link to the collective – the national tribe. As a result of this shift, Schwartz argues, the earlier model of trauma has to change because here it stops serving the purpose of understanding Appelfeld's work.

I would like to suggest that the trauma model is crucial to the experience that constitutes Appelfeld's personal, national, and poetic identity, and it nourishes the entire fabric of his literary works, including his later writing. Criticism should address shifts in the model, when necessary, but for an understanding of Appelfeld's works, I believe the trauma model should remain fundamental.

Poetic writing has the power to engage with and reflect internal reality, extricating the subject from the chaotic state of the traumatized self, on the brink of disintegration. By constructing the stages whereby poetic writing redeems individual trauma, I seek to establish a theoretical structure in which concepts from the domain of trauma explain the religious experience of communion with the world of the dead as part of a redemptive process, rather than as a shift away from the personal toward a tribal affinity. I propose that following extreme trauma, adherence to a transcendental state of mind, based on mystical-religious experience, is a stage leading to reconstitution of the self, including the poetic self.

Schwartz is not alone in reading Appelfeld within the broader context of Zionism or Judaism. Milner (2011), Hever (2017), and Oppenheimer (2014) consider Appelfeld's writing to hold out a "diasporist" alternative to hegemonic Zionist literature. Milner, writing about the story "Southern Sun,"[162] attempts to identify the story as a "diasporist" counter-narrative to the normative Zionist one. In my view, Appelfeld's writing is idiosyncratic, and where he touches on Zionism and Judaism this reflects his realistic autobiographical materials, without ideological import. He neither holds out an ideology nor does he propose to substitute one ideology with another.

La Capra[163] introduces the concept of *excess* in the discussion of extreme, traumatic events. There is, he argues, an excess at the heart of the traumatic experience, which escapes all representation and in this irrepresentability makes trauma present.[164] This excess can be identified in *The Man Who Never Stopped Sleeping*[165] as the liminal site of sleep. Sleep, it must be noted, is already mentioned in *Essays in the First Person*: "After years of drifting and suffering, Eretz Israel appeared a spaceous calming place which pulled one into a deep sleep. That exactly was the passion: to sleep, to be sleeping for years, become oblivious, and be born anew." This was a wonderful form of oblivion, Appelfeld said.[166]

The Man Who Never Stopped Sleeping starts with a description of the deep slumber into which Irwin has fallen:

> At the end of the war, I became immersed in constant slumber. Though I moved from train to train, from truck to truck, and sometimes from wagon to wagon, it was all in a dense, dreamless sleep [...] What happened to me during those days of sleep will probably be unknown to me forever [...].
>
> (p.3)

When asleep the boy dwells in deep oblivion of his trauma, in a hidden, inaccessible realm. Slumber is the liminal site at which the traumatic experience is registered, not owned, not processed and unrepresented in consciousness and language. This is the "excess" which can be experienced but not known; as Cathy Caruth's argues, this is a latency phase.[167]

Sleep in this novel constitutes a kind of placenta, a protective membrane enveloping the narrator until he will re-emerge into the world. Waking from sleep is described in terms of birth, being expelled from a protected place into blinding, wounding light (p.13). The involuntary departure from this protected space must of necessity involve the tearing of the placenta and is rendered as being caught up in a double-life. Though he is awake, the protagonist continues being nurtured by the darkness of slumber. When he is wounded in battle and is transferred to hospital, a new reality begins which transforms the nature of Irwin's sleep. Sleep in hospital becomes the space in which he matures toward creation, i.e., writing. When asleep the narrator sees people's faces more distinctly than ever before.

As he slowly recovers, slumber now is joined by preparation for writing the text "The First Home," a gradual awakening that takes the shape of the three versions Irwin writes before the final text. These versions are especially interesting because they correspond to the stages of processing the traumatic experience, which is being refined into the written text. The three drafts that appear in the novel are in fact early texts by Appelfeld which were published in their own right in Israeli periodicals.

Two of them, the first and the third, are poems (Appelfeld began his writing career as a poet,[168] and he published scores of poems in various journals between 1952 and 1959). This phenomenon, of a writer citing his own past work in later texts, I propose to call "auto-intertextuality."

Irwin's second draft consists of the opening of Appelfeld's short story "Slowly," which appeared in the short story collection *Smoke*, first published in 1962. This auto-intertextuality has the effect of creating an intended identity between author and his protagonist. Through this superposition, Appelfeld blurs the boundary between the author's writing and that of his protagonist, as the latter re-enacts the author's literary biography, repeating the author's early creation by using auto-intertextuality as a poetic device. The protagonist returns to the beginnings of the author's poetic biography. This journey toward the beginning in *The Man Who Never Stopped Sleeping* becomes Appelfeld-the-author's driving force on a journey that takes him through the boundaries of his own, actual life, toward former generations, through the limits of concrete reality to the beginnings of his biography as an artist.

Irwin's first draft includes a four-line poem. The first line marks the traumatic core, lack, lacuna, the unspeakable, unrepresented excess that remains locked within the pain, sealed with words welded in the furnace of suffering

That night, I wrote four lines:

> Not one word remains
> That wasn't refined in the furnace of pain.
> The storm is closed within me
> Behind bolted doors.

I revised them again and again, and I knew there was much more to revise. But my hands became fists, and I lay the pen down on the paper (pp.208–209).

The poem consists of a literal quote from the first strophe of Appelfeld's poem "Volcano" (*ga'ash*), which was published in the *Gazit* journal in 1957.[169]

The second draft is a quote from the short story "Slow," in the collection *Smoke* and it points at the invisible changes that occur in hidden processes. Development is slow and unnoticeable: it is halting, indirect and cryptic. This is what Appelfeld writes in *The Man Who Never Stopped Sleeping*:

> After a sleepless night […] I wrote the following lines at the first light:
>
> Unseen, the changes will come. Growth is slow, almost imperceptible. Only occasionally – at a station, at a temporary resting place, on a balcony – a face will peek out at you. It is encircled with wrinkles and, as on a sawed-off tree stump, you can count the rings of its years.
>
> I read it over and over. From where within me did those words sprout? And how had they joined together into a paragraph […] I was already beyond fatigue […] and I fell asleep.
>
> (p.224)

Here too, the draft mentioned in the novel reproduces an early stage of development in Appelfeld's poetic biography quoting part of the beginning of the short story mentioned above.

The third version again is a literal reiteration, this time of a stanza from an early poem by Appelfeld's, entitled "Now" (*ahshav*) published in 1957.[170] This quote provides the crack in the dam through which the writing pours. And it constitutes the moment before the religious revelation which becomes associated with the act of writing:

> That night I wrote the following lines:
> Now blood speaks.
> The caves spread, and the dams collapse.
> Now everything expects to be revealed
> In trembling.
> I felt a heavy pressure on my shoulders. [...] The four lines I had written were just a momentary opening into what was seeking to come into being.
> (*The Man Who Never Stopped Sleeping*, p.253)

From the void of trauma, the negative sublime, the lacuna, the inexpressible excess signaling the void left by trauma – an inaccessible, inconceivable and unrepresentable space, Appelfeld, undergoing a transcendental experience, turns his gaze toward the origin of his life and beyond, toward the lives of his parents, grandparents and great-grandparents.

Appelfeld's mode of connecting to the beginning is, chronologically speaking, in the *reverse – by turning back* to the origins of his family. By contrast, Haviva Pedaya, the cultural scholar, emphasizes, following Rabbi Kook, the *future* movement issuing from catastrophe, a sense of an ending which conceals the beginning of a new future.[171]

Appelfeld connects to this origin by looking back into his family's history. The Holy Sagi Nahor, Rabbi Michael, appears in his dreams and blesses him (pp.189, 216). In spite of its somewhat morbid, Orphean connotations, this offers access to the origins of their lives, for both Appelfeld and Irwin it. On thus returning to his ancestors, Appelfeld seems to break through the limits of time and space, traversing the generations beyond his own birth. Representational time of experience is a perpetual present, and the experience is a magical one, pure, simple, and crystal clear. Once the dam is burst, the redemptive moment arrives and writing surges forth:

> To return home. [...] usually in the hours of darkness [...] just then, a marvelous gate opens before you and invites you into your first home, your eternal home, which waits for you the way you left it.
> (p.265)

This journey to the origin is a driving force in Appelfeld's work. His journey traverses the boundaries of his own biological life, as well as his poetic biography. Writing about his origin becomes the site of religious experience enabling the re-creation of a lost world, the healing of torn connections, the restoring of voice to the mute. It is a revelation preceded by a long, slow, invisible process of consecration to writing.

Irwin's consecration to writing unfolds in two stages. The first is an intergenerational transmission whereby the father passes his pen to the protagonist, saying he can't do it anymore (p.93). The second goes beyond biology to a mythical reality through which the religious path unfolds: The protagonist is consecrated as a writer much like Samuel, Hannah's son, was anointed as a prophet (Samuel 1:1). It is the mother who is responsible for this mythical passage to the religious.[172] Consecration, in *The Man Who Never Stopped Sleeping*, occurs with the ritual of studying the first chapter of the Biblical book of Samuel with Slobotsky, the teacher. The story of Samuel's consecration projects by analogy onto the story of how Irwin, the protagonist, becomes a writer. The story of the protagonist's great-grandfather, Rabbi Michael Sagi Nahor, who appears in the protagonist's dream to bless him, is associated with one of the earliest Biblical narratives of consecration. These materials construct a narrative of consecration to prophecy that is transferred to the moment of the protagonist's turning writer.

Dedication to writing involves intensive training: Irwin mainly practices by copying from Genesis and Samuel, as well as from contemporary Hebrew literature like Agnon's stories. Copying brings him closer to the letters themselves, waiting to the day when the letters would be joined to his body and his voice (p.192). He expects that one day he will find his inner melody (p.207).

The First Home

In *The Man Who Never Stopped Sleeping*, the narrator makes a long journey toward his "first home," a journey that begins in the deep slumber of forgetting, continues through a double-life of wakefulness alongside sleep, and ends with autobiographical writing, constituting a narrative of retrospective redemption – not toward the afterlife, but in reverse, toward the origin. The "self" that has been unraveled by trauma is reconstituted by means of what preceded the traumatic experience, from within the abysmal origin that enables the poetic act of creation. The novel ends with the words of the frightened mother, warning him against the hazards of the journey, the cold regions and dangerous. She begs him to stay where he is and let the distant places come to him. Then she disappeared (p.287).

But Appelfeld is not Lot's wife who looks back at Sodom, and turns into a pillar of salt. Appelfeld, like *Gilgamesh*, who gazed into the abyss,[173] is the man who gazes into the abysmal origin, and from it he excavates a story of the reconstruction of a new and purified continuum, thus redeeming the disintegrated self.

Notes

1 Aharon Appelfeld, *Searing Light* [*Michvat Ha-Or*] (Hakibbutz Hameuchad, 1980). [Hebrew].

2 Aharon Appelfeld, *The Man Who Never Stopped Sleeping*, trans. Jeffrey M. Green (Schocken Books, [2010] 2017). Kindle Edition.

3 Shmuel Schneider, "Aharon Appelfeld on His Life and Works – An Interview", *Bitzaron 4* (1982), 5–17. [Hebrew].
4 Claudia Idan, "In the Human Image, A Conversation with the Author Aharon Appelfeld", *Pulmus 10* (1998), 41. [Hebrew].
5 Yaron Golan, "An Interview with Appelfeld", *Pi Ha'aton*, 5 May 1971. [Hebrew]; Moshe Singer, "Writing from Inside", *Hadoar*, 12 February 191. [Hebrew]; Schneider, "Aharon Appelfeld".
6 Yigal Schwartz, *The Individual's Lament and the Tribe's Eternity: Aharon Appelfeld – An Image of the World* (Magnes, 1996). [Hebrew].
7 Aharon Appelfeld, *Smoke* (Ahshav, 1962). [Hebrew].
8 Aharon Appelfeld, "Ongoing Bother", *Yediot Aharonot*, 10 December 1993.
9 Appelfeld, Smoke.
10 Schneider, "Aharon Appelfeld".
11 Appelfeld, "Ongoing Bother".
12 Yigal Schwartz, "Neither Apollo nor Alik – Interview", *Kol Ha'Ir*, 6 September 1991. [Hebrew].
13 Dan Laor, "Agnon, Appelfeld and the 'Jewish Myth'", *Haaretz*, 20 April 1995. [Hebrew].
14 Laor, "Agnon, Appelfeld and the 'Jewish Myth'".
15 Aharon Appelfeld, *Essays in the First Person* (The Zionist Library, 1979), 63. [Hebrew].
16 Appelfeld, *Essays in the First Person.*
17 Appelfeld, *Essays in the First Person*, 80, 86.
18 Aharon Appelfeld, *Iron Track* (Keter, 1991). [Hebrew].
19 Aharon Appelfeld, *The Ice Mine* (Keter, 1997). [Hebrew].
20 Aharon Appelfeld, *The Story of a Life*, trans. Aloma Halter (Shocken Books, [1999] 2004). Knopf Doubleday Publishing Group. Kindle Edition.
21 Appelfeld, *The Story of a Life*, 159, 162.
22 Appelfeld, *The Story of a Life*, 161.
23 Dan Miron, *Open Notebook: Discussions of Current Israeli Fiction* (Hapoalim, 1979). [Hebrew].
24 Miron, *Open Notebook*, 49–59.
25 Gershon Shaked, *A New Wave in Hebrew Fiction* (Sifriat Hapoalim, 1981), 71–86, 149–167. [Hebrew].
26 Shaked, *New Wave in Hebrew Fiction.*
27 Hillel Barzel, "Appelfeld's Affinity with Kafka", *Zehut 1* (1981), 112–120. [Hebrew].
28 See for instance, Natfali Tocker, "On *Searing Light* and the Terror of Shades", *Moznaim 52* (1981), 292–297. [Hebrew]; Gabriel Moked, "On *Searing Light*", *Al Hamishmar*, 1 October 1980. [Hebrew]; Yair Mazur, "The Writer's Song", *Aley Si'ah 23* (1986), 183–191. [Hebrew]; Lili Ratok, *Dangling Home* (Heker, 1989). [Hebrew]; Yigal Schwartz, "Poetics of Terror", *Davar*, 28 December 1979. [Hebrew]; Schwartz, *Individual's Lament*; Yigal Schwartz, *The Narrative Art of Aharon Appelfeld* (Dvir, 2014). [Hebrew]; Gila Ramraz-Ra'ukh, *Aharon Appelfeld: The Holocaust and Beyond* (Indiana UP, 1994).
29 See for example Michael Gluzman, "Memory and Blindness", *Mikan 5* (2005), 92–93, 97–98. [Hebrew].
30 Jochai Oppenheimer and Ketzia Allon, *Art and Symptom – Readings in Aharon Appelfeld* (Gamma, 2014), 18, 23. [Hebrew]; Hannan Hever, *We Are Fragments of Rhyme, Politics of Trauma in Israeli Literature* (Magnes, 2017), 106. [Hebrew].
31 Michael Gluzman, "So Far I Have Written the First Third – Interview with Aharon Appelfeld", *Mikan 1* (2000), 150–165. [Hebrew].

32 E.g., his comprehensive publications, *The Individual's Lament* and *Aharon Appelfeld's Art of Fiction.*
33 Yigal Schwartz, *Believer without a Church – Four Essays on Aharon Appelfeld* (Kineret, Zmoora Bitan, Dvir, 2009). [Hebrew].
34 Yigal Schwartz, "Preacher without Pulpit, Believer without Church: Aharon Appelfeld's Novel *Wild Blossoming*", in *Twenty-Four Readings in Aharon Appelfeld's Work*, eds. Avidov Lipsker and Avi Sagi (Bar Ilan University, 2011), 387. [Hebrew].
35 "Radioactive fallout" is a term Yolanda Gampel uses in her *Parents Who Live through Me* (Keter, 2010). [Hebrew].
36 Hever, *Fragments of Rhyme*, 106–107.
37 Rina Dudai, *Study of Devices Achieving an Effect of Restraint and Subtlety in a Charged Text* (MA dissertation, Tel Aviv University, 1983). [Hebrew]; Rina Dudai, *Modes of Coping with Trauma in Holocaust Literature (A. Appelfeld, Ka-tzetnik, P. Levi)* (doctoral dissertation, Hebrew University of Jerusalem, 2000). [Hebrew].
38 Dudai, *Modes of Coping.*
39 For a further development of these conceptualizations, see Schwartz, *Art of Fiction*, 122–128, on fictional space in Appelfeld's work.
40 John Lyons, *Semantics, Vol. 2* (Cambridge University Press, 1977), 638.
41 Lyons, *Semantics.*
42 Appelfeld, *Searing Light*, 10.
43 Appelfeld, *Searing Light*, 10.
44 Appelfeld, *Searing Light*, 18–19.
45 Appelfeld, *Searing Light*, 72–73.
46 Appelfeld, *Searing Light*, 73.
47 Cf. Schwartz's important article, "The Model of the Closed Camp: A Way Out?", *Siman Kriya 12–13* (1981), 357–360. [Hebrew].
48 Appelfeld, *Searing Light*, 155.
49 Appelfeld, *Searing Light*, 131.
50 Appelfeld, *Searing Light*, 119. [Here I changed pagination of quotes – RD].
51 Avraham Balaban, "The Big Problem Is How Not to Fake – An Interview with Aharon Appelfeld", *Yediot Aharonot*, 27 June 1980. [Hebrew].
52 Appelfeld, *Searing Light*, 122.
53 Appelfeld, *Searing Light*, 122.
54 Appelfeld, *Searing Light*, 122.
55 Appelfeld, *Searing Light*, 128.
56 Appelfeld, *Searing Light*, 7.
57 Appelfeld, *Searing Light*, 9.
58 Appelfeld, *Searing Light*, 106.
59 Appelfeld, *Searing Light*, 108.
60 Appelfeld, *Searing Light*, 108.
61 Appelfeld, *Searing Light*, 112.
62 Appelfeld, *Searing Light*, 113.
63 Appelfeld, *Searing Light*, 113.
64 William Labov, *Language in the Inner City: Studies in the Black English Vernacular* (University of Pennsylvania Press, 1972); Paul J. Hopper, "Aspect and Foregrounding in Discourse", in *Discourse and Syntax* (Academia Press, 1981), 211–241; Kurt Koffka, *Principles of Gestalt Psychology* (Harcourt, Brace, & World, 1963); Leonard Talmy, "Figure and Ground in Complex Sentences", *Annual Meeting of Berkeley Linguistics Society 1* (1975), 419–430.
65 Appelfeld, *Searing Light*, 139.
66 Appelfeld, *Searing Light*, 126.
67 Reuven Tsur, *What Is Cognitive Poetics?* (Tel Aviv University, 1982).

68 Appelfeld, *Searing Light*, 76.
69 Meyer H. Abrams, *A Glossary of Literary Terms* (Harcourt, Brace, 1993).
70 Lisa Silberstein, Howard Gardner, Erin Phelps, and Ellen Winner, "Autumn Leaves and Old Photographs: The Development of Metaphor", *Journal of Experimental Child Psychology 34:1* (1982), 135–150.
71 Appelfeld, *Searing Light*, 68–69.
72 Appelfeld, *Searing Light*, 122.
73 Appelfeld, *Searing Light*, 63.
74 Appelfeld, *Searing Light*, 109.
75 Dudai, *Study*, 1983.
76 John Lyons, "Deixis and Anaphora", in *The Development of Conversation and Discourse*, ed. Terry Myers (Edinburgh UP, 1979), 88–103.
77 Appelfeld, *Searing Light*, 150. From this point onward pagination of quoted text appears in body of text.
78 Here, I changed pagination system in order to emphasize the discontinuity between one sentence and the other.
79 Here I changed pagination system in order to emphasize the discontinuity between one sentence and the other.
80 Aristotle, *Poetics*, 8: 30–35, in *The Complete Works of Aristotle. The Revised Oxford Translation, Vol. 2*. ed. Jonathan Barnes (Princeton University Press, 1985), 2322.
81 Appelfeld, *Essays in the First Person*, 51–59.
82 Tzvetan Todorov, *The Poetics of Prose* (Cornell UP, 1977), 171.
83 Arnheim, in his book, discusses the distribution of centers throughout the entire work. He analyzes a painting by Mondrian, and I borrow his insight and use it to discuss the distribution of centers in the novel. Rudolf Arnheim, *The Power of the Center: A Study of Composition in the Visual Arts* (University of California Press, 1982), 2.
84 Arnheim offers quite a similar analysis in his above-mentioned work on Mondrian; *The Power*, 149–150.
85 Schwartz, "The Model of the Closed Camp"; Yigal Schwartz, *Aharon Appelfeld: From Individual Lament to Tribal Eternity*, trans. Jeffrey Green (Brandeis University Press, 2001); *The Narrative Art of Aharon Appelfeld* (Kinneret, Zmora-Bitan, Dvir, 2014) [Hebrew].
86 Schwartz, *Narrative Art*, 129.
87 Arnheim, *Power*, 150.
88 Barbara Herrnstein Smith, *Poetic Closure* (University of Chicago Press, 1974).
89 Herrnstein Smith, *Poetic Closure*, 100–102, 121, 188.
90 Silberstein et al., "Autumn Leaves".
91 Herrnstein Smith, *Poetic Closure*.
92 Rina Dudai, *Study of Devices Achieving an Effect of Restraint and Subtlety in a Charged Text*.
93 Elizabeth Brett and Robert Ostroff, "Imagery and Posttraumatic Stress Disorder: An Overview", *American Journal of Psychiatry 142:4* (1985), 417–424; Bessel A. Van der Kolk, *Psychological Trauma* (American Psychiatric Publishing, 1987); Bessel A. Van der Kolk and Onno Van der Hart, "The Intrusive Past: The Flexibility of Memory and the Engraving of Trauma", in *Trauma: Explorations in Memory*, ed. Cathy Caruth (The Johns Hopkins University Press, 1995), 158–182.
94 Allan Young, "Bodily Memory and Traumatic Memory", in *Tense Past: Cultural Essays in Trauma and Memory*, eds. Paul Antze and Michael Lambek (Routledge, 1996), 99.
95 Young, "Bodily Memory", 97.
96 Pnina Maiseles, "An Hour with Aharon Appelfeld", *Haboker*, 10 July 1964. [Hebrew].
97 Appelfeld, *Essays in the First Person*, 95.

98 Appelfeld, *Essays in the First Person*, 96.
99 Shin Shifra, "The Ability to Live and the Ability to Forget", An Interview with Aharon Appelfeld. *Massa*, 24 October, 1975.
100 Appelfeld, "Ongoing Bother".
101 Appelfeld, *The Story of a Life*, 168–169.
102 Appelfeld, *Essays in the First Person*, 48.
103 Idan, "In the Human Image", 42.
104 Schwartz, "Neither Apollo".
105 Schwartz, *Art of the Story*, 28.
106 Jean-François Lyotard, "Anamnesis: Of the Visible", *Theory, Culture and Society 21* (2004), 107–119.
107 Aharon Appelfeld, *The Age of Wonders* (Hakibbutz Hameuchad, 1978). [Hebrew].
108 Schwartz, *Art of the* Story, 68.
109 Appelfeld, *Essays in the First Person*. [Hebrew].
110 Edna Evron, "Aharon Appelfeld – Total Writer", *Yediot Aharonot*, 17 June 1994. [Hebrew].
111 Appelfeld, *The Story of a Life*, 114.
112 Aharon Appelfeld, *All Whom I Have Loved* (Schocken, 2007), 25.
113 Appelfeld, *All Whom I Have Loved*, 212.
114 Evron, "Aharon Appelfeld".
115 Shulamith Gingold-Gilboa, "Aharon Appelfed", *Iton 77:46* (1983), 28–29. [Hebrew].
116 Appelfeld, *The Story of a Life*, 97.
117 Julia Kristeva, *Revolution in Poetic Language*, trans. Margaret Waller (Columbia UP, 1984).
118 Appelfeld, *The Man Who Never Stopped Sleeping*.
119 Kristeva, *Revolution.*
120 Julia Kristeva, *New Maladies of the Soul*, trans. Ross Guberman (Columbia UP, 1995) 31–33.
121 Dylan Evans, *An Introductory Dictionary of Lacanian Psychoanalysis* (Routledge, 1996).
122 Kristeva, *Revolution.*
123 Kristeva, *Revolution.*
124 Shin Shifra, "The Ability to Live – The Ability to Forget" (interview) *Davar*, 1975. [Hebrew].
125 Aharon, Appelfeld, "Ongoing Bother", *Yediot Aharonot*, 10 December 1993. [Hebrew].
126 Aharon Appelfeld, "A Talk on the Occasion of Being Awarded the Ussishkin Prize, 1966", *Am Ve'Admato*, January 1967, 21–22.
127 From an interview with Anat Levit; Anat Levit, "Interview with Aharon Appelfeld", *Davar*, 10 January 1986. [Hebrew].
128 Aharon Appelfeld, *All Whom I Have Loved* (Schocken, 2007).
129 Aharon Appelfeld, *The Journey into Winter* (Keter, 2000). [Hebrew].
130 Appelfeld, *Essays in the First Person*, 67–68.
131 Dan Miron, "Open Notebook", *Haaretz*, 6 March 1964. [Hebrew]; Gershon Shaked, "The Force of Survival", *Yediot Aharonot*, 8 January 1984. [Hebrew].
132 Edna Evron, "Aharon Appelfeld – Total Writer", *Yediot Achronot*, 17 June 1994. [Hebrew].
133 Yigal Schwartz, "Neither Apollo nor Alik – Interview", *Kol Ha'Ir*, 6 September 1991. [Hebrew].
134 Rachel Albeck-Gidron, "The Lexicon and the Flood", in *Twenty-Four Readings*, eds. Avidov Lipsker and Avi Sagi (Bar Ilan University, 2011), 153. [Hebrew].
135 Evron, "Aharon Appelfeld".
136 Appelfeld, *The Man Who Never Stopped Sleeping*.

137 Peter Haidu, "The Dialectics of Unspeakability: Language, Silence, and the Narratives of Desubjectification", in *Probing the Limits of Representation*, ed. Saul Friedlander (Harvard UP, 1993), 283–284; Dominick LaCapra, *Representing the Holocaust* (Cornell UP, 1996), 105; Dominick LaCapra, *History and Memory after Auschwitz* (Cornell UP, 1998), 38; Berel Lang, *Act and Idea in the Nazi Genocide* (Chicago UP, 1990), 161.
138 Haviva Pedaya, *Going beyond Trauma* (Resling, 2011), 22. [Hebrew].
139 Yigal Schwartz, *Aharon Appelfeld: From Individual Lament to Tribal Eternity* (Brandeis University Press, 2001).
140 Yigal Schwartz, *Aharon Appelfeld's Art of Fiction* (Dvir, 2014). [Hebrew Edition].
141 Schwartz, *Aharon Appelfeld's Art of Fiction*, 158.
142 Schwartz, *Aharon Appelfeld's Art of Fiction*, 162. See also, Zahava Caspi, "Removing the Peel and Revealing the Core", *Mikan 5* (2005), 47–56. [Hebrew].
143 Appelfeld, *Essays in the First Person*, 62.
144 Edmund Burke, *A Philosophical Enquiry* (Oxford UP, 1990).
145 Jean-François Lyotard, *The Postmodern Condition*, trans. Geoff Bennington and Brian Massumi (Minneapolis UP, 1993); Jean-François Lyotard, *Lessons on the Analytic of the Sublime*, trans. Elizabeth Rottenberg (Stanford UP, 1994).
146 Burke, *Philosophical Enquiry*, 54–55.
147 Burke, *Philosophical Enquiry*, 125–126.
148 Lyotard, *Postmodern Condition*, 78.
149 Appelfeld, *Essays in the First Person*, 98.
150 Jean Améry, *At the Mind's Limits: Contemplation by a Survivor on Auschwitz and Its Realities*, trans. Sidney Rosenfeld and Stella P. Rosenfeld (Indiana University Press, 2009).
151 Améry, *At the Mind's Limits*, 69–70.
152 Appelfeld, *Essays in the First Person*, 71.
153 Appelfeld, *Essays in the First Person*, 25.
154 Burke, *Philosophical Enquiry*, 62–63.
155 See also Iris Milner, who points out religious experience in Appelfeld's work as an expression of an intimate affinity with God; Iris Milner, "On 'the Language in Which We Talk with God' – A Politics of Space and Drifting", in *Twenty-Four Readings* in Aharon Appelfeld's Work, eds. Avidov Lipsker and Avi Sagi (Bar Ilan University, 2011), 480. [Hebrew].
156 Appelfeld, *Essays in the First Person*, 98.
157 Appelfeld, *Essays in the First Person*, 99.
158 Paul Antze and Michael Lambek, eds., *Tense Past* (Routledge, 1996); Young, "Bodily Memory and Traumatic Memory", 89–102.
159 Appelfeld, *The Man Who Never Stopped Sleeping*.
160 For a shorter version: Rina Dudai, "From Excess to Origin: Traversing Time Zones as an Act of Redemption in the 'Man Who Never Stopped Sleeping' by Aharon Appelfeld", *Yod. Revue des etudes hebraiques and juives 19* (2014), 249–258.
161 Yigal Schwartz, "Preacher without Pulpit, Believer without Church: Aharon Appelfeld's Novel Wild Blossoming", in Avidov Lipsker and Avi Sagi, eds., *Twenty-Four Readings in Aharon Appelfeld's Work* (Bar Ilan University, 2011), 387. [Hebrew].
162 Milner, "On 'the Language in Which We Talk with God'".
163 Dominick LaCapra, *Writing History, Writing Trauma* (Johns Hopkins University Press, 2000). [Hebrew Edition 2006].
164 LaCapra, *Writing History*, 15, 50, 119–121.
165 Appelfeld, *The Man Who Never Stopped Sleeping*. References from this point onwards will appear in the body of the text.
166 Appelfeld, *Essays in the First Person*, 35, 37. [Hebrew].

167 Cathy Caruth, *Unclaimed Experience* (Johns Hopkins UP, 1996), 16–18.
168 See Schwartz on this phase in Appelfeld's writing life: *Aharon Appelfeld: From Individual Lament to Tribal Eternity* (Brandeis University Press, 2001), 144.
169 Aharon Appelfeld, "Gaash", *Gazit 14* (1957), 20. [Hebrew].
170 Aharon Appelfeld, "Now", *Gazit 15* (1957), 30. [Hebrew].
171 Pedaya, *Going beyond Trauma*, 581–582, 599, 622. [Hebrew].
172 See also Milner, who identifies the close approach to God with a consoling maternal space. In Iris Milner, "Following the Language One Talks with God", in *Twenty-Four Readings in Aharon Appelfeld's Literary Work*, eds. Avidov Lipsker and Avi Sagi (Bar-Ilan University Press, 2011), 467–488.
173 Shin Shifra and Jacob Klein, eds., *In Those Distant Days: Anthology of Mesopotamian Literature in Hebrew* (Am Oved, [1996], 2010), 185. [Hebrew].

References

Abrams, Meyer H., *A Glossary of Literary Terms* (Harcourt, Brace & World, 1993).

Albeck-Gidron, Rachel, "The Lexicon and the Flood", in Avidov Lipsker and Avi Sagi, eds., *Twenty-Four Readings* (Bar Ilan University, 2011), 153–161. [Hebrew].

Améry, Jean, *At the Mind's Limits: Contemplation by a Survivor on Auschwitz and Its Realities*, trans. Sidney Rosenfeld and Stella P. Rosenfeld (Indiana University Press, 2009).

Antze, Paul and Lambek, Michael, eds., *Tense Past: Cultural Essays in Trauma and Memory* (Routledge, 1996).

Appelfeld, Aharon, "Gaash", *Gazit 14* (1957), 20. [Hebrew].

Appelfeld, Aharon, "Now", *Gazit 15* (1957), 30. [Hebrew].

Appelfeld, Aharon, *Smoke* (Ahshav, 1962). [Hebrew].

Appelfeld, Aharon, "A Talk on the Occasion of Being Awarded the Ussishkin Prize, 1966", *Am Ve'Admato*, January 1967.

Appelfeld, Aharon, *The Age of Wonders* (Hakibbutz Hameuchad, 1978). [Hebrew].

Appelfeld, Aharon, *Essays in the First Person* (The Zionist Library, 1979), 63. [Hebrew].

Appelfeld, Aharon, *Searing Light* [*Michvat Ha-Or*] (Hakibbutz Hameuchad, 1980). [Hebrew].

Appelfeld, Aharon, *Iron Track* (Keter, 1991). [Hebrew].

Appelfeld, Aharon, "Ongoing Bother", *Yediot Aharonot*, 10 December 1993.

Appelfeld, Aharon, *The Ice Mine* (Keter, 1997). [Hebrew].

Appelfeld, Aharon, *The Story of a Life*, trans. Aloma Halter (Shocken Books, [1999] 2004). Knopf Doubleday Publishing Group. Kindle Edition.

Appelfeld, Aharon, *The Journey into Winter* (Keter, 2000). [Hebrew].

Appelfeld, Aharon, *All Whom I Have Loved* (Schocken, 2007).

Appelfeld, Aharon, *The Man Who Never Stopped Sleeping*, trans. Jeffrey M. Green (Schocken Books, [2010] 2017). Kindle Edition.

Aristotle, *Poetics*, 8: 30–35, in *The Complete Works of Aristotle. The Revised Oxford Translation, Vol. 2*. ed. Jonathan Barnes (Princeton University Press, 1985), 2322.

Arnheim, Rudolf, *The Power of the Center: A Study of Composition in the Visual Arts* (University of California Press, 1982).

Balaban, Avraham, "The Big Problem Is How Not to Fake – An Interview with Aharon Appelfeld", *Yediot Aharonot*, 27 June 1980. [Hebrew].

Barzel, Hillel, "Appelfeld's Affinity with Kafka", *Zehut 1* (1981), 112–120. [Hebrew].

Brett, Elizabeth and Ostroff, Robert, "Imagery and Posttraumatic Stress Disorder: An Overview", *American Journal of Psychiatry 142:4* (1985), 417–424.

Burke, Edmund, *A Philosophical Enquiry* (Oxford UP, [1757],1990).

Caruth, Cathy, ed., *Trauma: Explorations in Memory* (The Johns Hopkins University Press, 1995).

Caruth, Cathy, *Unclaimed Experience* (Johns Hopkins UP, 1996).

Caspi, Zahava, "Removing the Peel and Revealing the Core", *Mikan 5* (2005) 47–56. [Hebrew].

Dudai, Rina, *Study of Devices Achieving an Effect of Restraint and Subtlety in a Charged Text* (MA dissertation, Tel Aviv University, 1983). [Hebrew].

Dudai, Rina, *Modes of Coping with Trauma in Holocaust Literature (A. Appelfeld, Katzetnik, P. Levi)* (doctoral dissertation, Hebrew University of Jerusalem, 2000). [Hebrew].

Dudai, Rina, "From Excess to Origin: Traversing Time Zones as an Act of Redemption in the 'Man Who Never Stopped Sleeping' by Aharon Appelfeld", *Yod. Revue des etudes hebraiques and juives 19* (2014), 249–258.

Evron, Edna, "Aharon Appelfeld – Total Writer", *Yediot Aharonot*, 17 June 1994. [Hebrew].

Gampel, Yolanda, *Parents Who Live through Me* (Keter, 2010). [Hebrew].

Gingold-Gilboa, Shulamith, "Aharon Appelfed", *Iton 77:46* (1983), 28–29. [Hebrew].

Gluzman, Michael, "So Far I Have Written the First Third – Interview with Aharon Appelfeld", *Mikan 1* (2000), 150–165. [Hebrew].

Gluzman, Michael, "Memory and Blindness", *Mikan 5* (2005), 92–93, 97–98. [Hebrew].

Golan, Yaron, "An Interview with Appelfeld", *Pi Ha'aton*, 5 May 1971. [Hebrew]; Moshe Singer, "Writing from Inside", *Hadoar*, 12 February 191. [Hebrew].

Haidu, Peter, "The Dialectics of Unspeakability: Language, Silence, and the Narratives of Desubjectification", in Saul Friedlander, ed., *Probing the Limits of Representation* (Harvard UP, 1993), 283–284.

Herrnstein Smith, Barbara, *Poetic Closure* (University of Chicago Press, 1974).

Hever, Hannan, *We Are Fragments of Rhyme, Politics of Trauma in Israeli Literature* (Magnes, 2017), 106. [Hebrew].

Hopper, Paul J., "Aspect and Foregrounding in Discourse", in Talmy Givon, ed., *Discourse and Syntax* (Academia Press, 1981), 211–241.

Idan, Claudia, "In the Human Image, a Conversation with the Author Aharon Appelfeld", *Pulmus 10* (1998), 41. [Hebrew].

Koffka, Kurt, *Principles of Gestalt Psychology* (Harcourt, Brace & World, 1963).

Kristeva, Julia, *Revolution in Poetic Language*, trans. Margaret Waller (Columbia UP, 1984).

Kristeva, Julia, *New Maladies of the Soul*, trans. Ross Guberman (Columbia UP, 1995).

Labov, William, *Language in the Inner City: Studies in the Black English Vernacular* (University of Pennsylvania Press, 1972).

LaCapra, Dominick, *Representing the Holocaust* (Cornell UP, 1996).

LaCapra, Dominick, *History and Memory after Auschwitz* (Cornell UP, 1998).

Lang, Berel, *Act and Idea in the Nazi Genocide* (Chicago UP, 1990).

Laor, Dan, "Agnon, Appelfeld and the 'Jewish Myth'", *Haaretz*, 20 April 1995. [Hebrew].

Levit, Anat, "Interview with Aharon Appelfeld", *Davar*, 10 January 1986. [Hebrew].

Lipsker, Avidov and Sagi, Avi, eds., *Twenty-Four Readings in Aharon Appelfeld's Work* (Bar Ilan University, 2011). [Hebrew].

Lyons, John, *Semantics, Vol. 2* (Cambridge University Press, 1977).

Lyons, John, "Deixis and Anaphora", in Terry Myers, ed., *The Development of Conversation and Discourse* (Edinburgh UP, 1979), 88–103.

Lyotard, Jean-François, *The Postmodern Condition*, trans. Geoff Bennington and Brian Massumi (Minneapolis UP, 1993).
Lyotard, Jean-François, *Lessons on the Analytic of the Sublime*, trans. Elizabeth Rottenberg (Stanford UP, 1994).
Lyotard, Jean-François, "Anamnesis: Of the Visible", *Theory, Culture and Society 21* (2004), 107–119.
Maiseles, Pnina, "An Hour with Aharon Appelfeld", *Haboker*, 10 July 1964. [Hebrew].
Mazur, Yair, "The Writer's Song", *Aley Si'ah 23* (1986), 183–191. [Hebrew].
Milner, Iris, "On 'the Language in which we Talk with God' – A Politics of Space and Drifting", in Avidov Lipsker and Avi Sagi, eds., *Twenty-Four Readings in Aharon Appelfeld's Work* (Bar Ilan University, 2011), 467–488. [Hebrew].
Miron, Dan, *Open Notebook: Discussions of Current Israeli Fiction* (Hapoalim, 1979). [Hebrew].
Moked, Gabriel, "On *Searing Light*" *Al Hamishmar*, 1 October 1980. [Hebrew].
Oppenheimer, Jochai and Allon, Ketzia, *The Art and Symptom – Reading Aharon Appelfeld* (Gamma, 2014), 18, 23. [Hebrew].
Ovid, *Metamorphosis*, trans. A.S. Kline, IV:753–803; Perseus Tells the Story of Medusa. Poetryintranslation.com (2000).
Pedaya, Haviva, *Going beyond Trauma* (Resling, 2011), 22. [Hebrew].
Ramraz-Ra'ukh, Gila, *Aharon Appelfeld: The Holocaust and Beyond* (Indiana UP, 1994).
Ratok, Lili, *Dangling Home* (Heker, 1989). [Hebrew].
Schneider, Shmuel, "Aharon Appelfeld on His Life and Works – An Interview", *Bitzaron 4* (1982), 5–17. [Hebrew].
Schwartz, Yigal, "Poetics of Terror", *Davar*, 28 December 1979. [Hebrew].
Schwartz, Yigal, "The Model of the Closed Camp: A Way Out?", *Siman Kriya 12–13* (1981), 357–360. [Hebrew].
Schwartz, Yigal, "Neither Apollo nor Alik – Interview", *Kol Ha'Ir*, 6 September 1991. [Hebrew].
Schwartz, Yigal, *Aharon Appelfeld: From Individual Lament to Tribal Eternity*, trans. Jeffrey Green (Brandeis University Press, 2001).
Schwartz, Yigal, *Believer without a Church – Four Essays on Aharon Appelfeld* (Kineret, Zmoora Bitan, Dvir, 2009). [Hebrew].
Schwartz, Yigal, "Preacher without Pulpit, Believer without Church: Aharon Appelfeld's Novel *Wild Blossoming*", in Avidov Lipsker and Avi Sagi, eds., *Twenty-Four Readings in Aharon Appelfeld's Work* (Bar Ilan University, 2011), 387. [Hebrew].
Schwartz, Yigal, *The Narrative Art of Aharon Appelfeld* (Kinneret, Zmora-Bitan, Dvir, 2014). [Hebrew].
Shaked, Gershon, *A New Wave in Hebrew Fiction* (Sifriat Hapoalim, 1981), 71–86, 149–167. [Hebrew].
Shaked, Gershon, "The Force of Survival", *Yediot Aharonot*, 8 January 1984. [Hebrew].
Shifra, Shin, "The Ability to Live and the Ability to Forget", An Interview with Aharon Appelfeld. *Davar*, 24 October, 1975.
Shifra, Shin and Jacob, Klein, eds., *In Those Distant Days: Anthology of Mesopotamian Literature in Hebrew* (Am Oved, [1996], 2010), 185. [Hebrew].
Silberstein, Lisa, Gardner, Howard, Phelps, Erin, and Winner, Ellen, "Autumn Leaves and Old Photographs: The Development of Metaphor", *Journal of Experimental Child Psychology 34:1* (1982), 135–150.

Singer, Moshe, "Writing from Inside", *Hadoar*, 12 February 191. [Hebrew].
Talmy, Leonard, "Figure and Ground in Complex Sentences", *Annual Meeting of Berkeley Linguistics Society 1* (1975), 419–430.
Tocker, Natfali, "On *Searing Light* and the Terror of Shades", *Moznaim 52* (1981), 292–297. [Hebrew].
Todorov, Tzvetan, *The Poetics of Prose* (Cornell UP, 1977).
Tsur, Reuven, *What Is Cognitive Poetics?* (Tel Aviv University, 1982).
Van der Kolk, Bessel A., *Psychological Trauma* (American Psychiatric Publishing, 1987).
Van der Kolk, Bessel A. and Van der Hart, Onno, "The Intrusive Past: The Flexibility of Memory and the Engraving of Trauma", in Caruth Cathy, ed., *Trauma: Explorations in Memory* (The Johns Hopkins University Press, 1995), 158–182.
Young, Allan, "Bodily Memory and Traumatic Memory", in Paul Antze and Michael Lambek, eds., *Tense Past: Cultural Essays in Trauma and Memory* (Routledge, 1996), 99.

Chapter 4

On Emotional Traumatic Memory in Ka-Tzetnik's *The House of Dolls*[1]

> Like everybody else, I also believed that no one could pass through this cataclysm of fire and come out alive. This, perhaps, was why I always pushed myself right into the forefront of danger: So the pupils of my eyes would film the scenes. Maybe one day, someone would find my eyes, whole and unburnt, to discover in them final testimony of the horror I witnessed.[2]

Yehiel Dinur (Feiner), the Man Who Screams His Testimony[3]

In the above quotation, Dinur presents us with one condensed expression concerning his place in relation to traumatic experience: Following a "cataclysm of fire" – a mythological event involving a deluge of water and fire – only his eye survives as a metonymic remainder of a disintegrated whole. The eye, which the author compares to a film camera, turns into an autonomous object which mechanically documents everything it faces. The registering eye can only do its job if the person whose eye it is puts himself right at the forefront, in the way of the dangerous fire flood, where the most horrific spectacle unfolds. Though the owner of the eye may perish, the camera that is his eye will survive, with the filmed material intact. One day, these materials will be unearthed like archeological finds: final testimony to the horror.

This is how Dinur presents himself to the world: the owner of a bionic-mythological eye who dedicates his life to giving documentary testimony. He understands the act of witnessing as mandatory and objectively true. The eye has no choice but to film, and it acquits itself of its task with the faithfulness of an actual camera. Even as everything else goes up in the flames of horror, the eye, unharmed, will testify. The speaker commits to self-abnegation in the face of this mythical reality. Dinur will focus on documenting the observed reality rather than on the observer, on the camera's mechanical eye rather than on the interpreting eye, which renders subjective interpretation and insight.

The author took to the witness stand in session number 68 of the Eichmann trial, in Jerusalem, on 7 June 1961, to testify about Auschwitz. When asked for his true

DOI: 10.4324/9781003403753-7

name, he said: "Yehiel Dinur." When asked to explain his literary pseudonym, Ka-Tzetnik, he responded with these, often quoted, words:

> It isn't a pen name. I don't think of myself as a writer of literary fiction. It's a chronicle from Planet Auschwitz. I was there, for about two years. Time there is unlike time here, on Earth. Every fraction of a second, there, unfolds from a different wheel. The people who inhabited that planet did not carry names. They had neither parents nor children. They did not dress in the manner familiar to us. They were not born there nor did they give birth. Their breathing was subject to different laws of nature. They neither lived nor died according to the rules that this world here goes by. Their name was a number: Ka-Tzetnik [concentration camp inmate]. They wore no name.[4]

The presiding judge intervened, and Dinur rose, stepped down from the witness stand, and collapsed. The session was interrupted.[5] Dinur was hospitalized.

Changing one's name is no small matter. Dinur did not alter his private name to any other private name; he substituted it with a general name – Ka-Tzetnik, literally: concentration camp inmate – detaching himself from his personal identity. He thereby included himself in the mass of people who turned into a nameless entity and whose representative he felt called to be. His is an act of self-denial in the face of the collective perished camp prisoners. During the one public event in which he could give expression to these two commitments, he fainted and collapsed. Intended to represent the murdered millions, his testimony folded as he fell to the floor, failing to be passed on. The courtroom exposed Dinur to the actual world, without defense mechanisms. What was left, in such a context, was silence. In fainting, Dinur staked out the limits of discourse. To the prosecutor, defense attorney, judges, president of the court, and the assembled witnesses and audience, he was a reminder that the formal discourse of the law is not always appropriate to the intensity of the catastrophic experience which is essentially beyond words. Dinur had chosen to give his account as an artist who renders his outcry through literature rather than in the actual reality of the courtroom.[6]

Yehiel Dinur, a Short Biography

Yehiel Dinur (Feiner) was born in 1909 to a traditional Jewish family in Sosnowiec, in Poland, a city on the border between Silesia and Galicia in a region dominated by the mining industry. He studied at the Lublin Yeshiva and was a member of the Orthodox Jewish "Agudat Yisrael Youth." Before the war, his poetry in Yiddish and Hebrew had been published in the Sosnowiec Revisionist publication *Unser Tagblat*,[7] in *Das Yiddishe Wokhenblat*, which came out in Warsaw, and in the Hebrew-language monthly *Darkenu*.[8] He was 22 when he published a book of poetry in Yiddish.[9] Following the Nazi occupation, he first lived in the Katowice ghetto until he was put on transport to Auschwitz, where he spent, as mentioned, about two years. After liberation, he reached a British military base in Naples, Italy, as part of a joint Jewish Brigade and Haganah action. There he withdrew into a room, writing *Salamandra* in the course of two and a half weeks, the first part of a family story he called "A Chronicle of a Jewish Family in the 20th Century."[10]

The name Ka-Tzetnik derives from the German acronym for concentration camp: *Konzentrationslager*, abbreviated as KZ (and pronounced *ka-tzet*). The soldier to whom Ka-Tzetnik eventually handed over the manuscript was Eliyahu Goldenberg, an actor from the Jewish Yishuv in Palestine, who passed it on to Zalman Rubashov (better known as Shazar, eventually Israel's third president), and he in turn gave it to I.D. Berkowitz, the writer and translator. Berkowitz translated the Yiddish text into Hebrew, and it was published by Dvir in 1946,[11] even before Dinur himself reached Palestine.[12]

Ka-Tzetnik published more books, originally in Hebrew, following this novel: *Beit Habubot* (1953; Eng. *House of Dolls*, 1955); *Piepel* (1961; Eng. *Piepel*, 1961); *Hasha'on* (1960; Eng. *The Clock*, 1966); *Ha'imut* (1966; Eng. *The Confrontation*, 1969); *Ha'tsofen* (1987; Eng. *The Code*, or *Shivitti*, 1989). These books all describe the author's experience in the concentration camp, the story of his relatives' fate: his sister, his brother and sister-in-law, who all perished, as well as his struggle for a new life in Israel.[13]

Years after the Eichmann trial, Dinur underwent unconventional post-trauma treatment, which included the supervised use of LSD. His book *The Code* records this experience. When in the course of an LSD-induced hallucination, he saw himself in an SS uniform, wearing the infamous cap with the skull symbol, and he realized that both victim and perpetrator were human beings who might find themselves in opposite roles. He stopped the treatment, stating that he had suffered from nightmares before the therapy, while after it, these dreams also attacked him when awake.[14] Ka-Tzetnik died in July 2001.

Becoming Publicly Known

Ka-Tzetnik's literary howl inaugurated a process of collective mourning in Israel. A loud, primal scream was needed to burst through public defenses. Miron described how violently Ka-Tzetnik's books, deploying their cheap literary effects, struck his Israeli readership. Only in this way could he penetrate a public consciousness deeply immersed in the project of building a new society. Miron believed that Ka-Tzetnik's books, in that sense, broke through an imposed silence.[15]

Miron examines what he considers the naturalistic character of Ka-Tzetnik's concrete images. These images are direct, provocative, and stunning, but, he argues, due to the mythic-ideological, anti-historical, and anti-psychological interpretation of their subject matter, they impose a simplistic view on an extremely complex reality.

The importance of Ka-Tzetnik's work, according to the critics, was in how it reconstructed the memory of the trauma, its capacity to touch the very heart of the matter and represent it, thereby anchoring it in the collective memory.

A fellow Auschwitz survivor of Ka-Tzetnik writes:

> The descriptions give us no respite…and it is true. That's exactly why they were written: so, we will have no respite. For the pain is terrible, the disaster great, and we are obliged not to forget it through many generations.[16]

The powerful reaction Ka-Tzetnik stirred in many of his readers is based on his realistic, naturalistic writing, which manages to enact this traumatic memory right before their eyes. Many of his readers said it felt like looking at painting or photography: "This is no ordinary writing: it is neither diary nor fiction. What we have is a painting, right before our very eyes; there's a description of sounds and voices to experience again, in our very body and mind."[17] And this is another critic: "Ka-Tzetnik is not a mere story-teller, but a master painter, whose words evoke colors, as he describes a landscape and mood, stirrings of the soul and its loneliness." And, "If any literary work … can be expected to show the reader what happened, it is Ka-Tzetnik's oeuvre… It touches the raw, living flesh, the thing that scalds, the fire itself."[18] K.A. Bertini uses the image of a relief rather than a painting or photograph:

> The book is powerful in adding its very own expression of the manifold horrors of the Holocaust. The images, no, I'd rather call them reliefs, are deep engravings, as if a nail had been cutting into the flesh. … And these reliefs are stunning. … Here's the whip, and here the rusty tin into which soup was poured…Here are the chairs of those sentenced to 'purification', and here the trucks loaded with frozen corpses….[19]

The reader becomes an actual witness to the atrocities.[20] Some readers reported a sense of oppression and coercion: "One cannot read these two books without feeling shocked."[21] "Once one has read a book of his it is impossible to get rid of the scenes and states of mind they describe."[22] "His descriptions are hypnotic, pouring their poison insistently."[23] "The author forcefully imposes this morbidity, with the effect, once you've read it, […] you feel as though you had been there yourself, and that you're really one of those who were miraculously saved."[24]

> Ka-Tzetnik, the author of *House of Dolls*, has the gift to remove us from our reality with its abundantly clear skies … yearnings for freedom and patriotic vision, and force upon us a world of murder, stupidity and baseness…We are dragged into this world, we find ourselves delivered to it by sentences made up out of letters, recounted facts, people who come and go.[25]

The effect on readers was so powerful we might call it a second-order post-traumatic reaction. Critics and regular readers alike reported feelings of helplessness and profound shock, as well as physiological reactions like palpitations, sleep disturbances, and shortness of breath. This is Yotam Reuveni:

> I read *Salamandra* and constantly wanted to stop and escape. I experienced a strange sense of fragmentation, diffusion: The death, madness, senselessness of what went on in Auschwitz kept coming at me, but I moved away, dwelling on passages where the madness wasn't so absolute... *Salamandra* is a scary book. It is about helpless people and the reader, too, feels helpless.[26]

And here is what Yeshurun Keshet wrote about *House of Dolls*:

> A terrifying, oppressing book which engraves itself indelibly. One's heart, full of misgivings, pounds, contracts and misses a beat, like when someone hurts your feelings and you're defenseless and cannot prove you're right, because there are no words in your mouth and your throat chokes.[27]
>
> I read the book for weeks because after the torture of reading those descriptions ... I couldn't sleep at night.[28]

Emanuel Ben-Gurion reported actual post-traumatic symptoms after reading *House of Dolls*:

> After reading *House of Dolls*, you find yourself walking among your fellow citizens, stunned – the streets appear cheerful, boys and girls at play...All of a sudden, a flash of anxiety strikes: This quiet, peaceful scene of innocence and joy, beauty and liveliness... is it really nothing but an illusion? And you realize you will never again be able to look at this Jewish girl, your student, or your son's girlfriend, or just some passerby, as before, with a sincere, human gaze. You see her differently, from a different perspective, her body carrying the tattoo.[29]

The author arouses readers' intense emotion by resurrecting the atrocities. This in turn entails a kind of textual acting-out, whose materials – while being poetically wrapped – have an amplifying effect.[30] *House of Dolls* was Israeli readers' first encounter with a description of an extermination camp, fully exposing the atrocities.

Ka-Tzetnik's readership dwindled over the years, though he stayed relatively popular among the young: his work is still on the official school curriculum. Omer Bartov argued that Israeli youth, prior to 1967, had access to two types of Holocaust literature: "legitimate" and "illegitimate."[31] The first category consisted of the heroic literature, which, he claimed, features Jews who participated in ghetto uprisings and includes them in the Zionist pantheon. The "illegitimate" type of literature consisted of so-called "Stalag" books, popular in the 1960s, pornographic paperbacks teeming with sex and sadism, whose narratives were situated in the camps. These books circulated secretly between young readers, out of the adults' sight. The genre was part of the non-formal sexual education of Israeli teenagers of that period.

Bartov argued that *House of Dolls* straddled the boundary between these "legitimate" and "illegitimate" texts. The book does not glorify resistance in the characteristic way of the legitimate genre, yet its descriptions of physical and mental horrors are not strictly pornographic. For Bartov, Ka-Tzetnik's Holocaust descriptions were unprecedented in the Holocaust literature due to their daring rendering of such charged material and in an immature, banal literary style.[32] More recently scholars have returned to Ka-Tzetnik's work as a successful attempt at an unfiltered description of life in the camps. Most of this work, however, is historical, treating the author's work as documentation rather than considering its poetics as an attempt to render his experience in a way that would prompt his readers' identification.

The Scream: The Personal Urge to Write

Behind Ka-Tzetnik's obsessive urge to make contact with trauma and to record it in writing, a vocation was felt: a commitment to represent an absent collective or to represent memory for a collective of survivors. At the same time, his obsessive writing can also be considered in terms of the personal processing of trauma, a form of processing that may have significant implications also for the collective memory. The present reading of Ka-Tzetnik's literary testimony does not only concern the literary-poetic representation of trauma or the transmission of historical data: it also looks at the survivor's processing of trauma.[33]

Trauma processing involves mourning about a past that refuses to be forgotten, a past that insists on its right of return. The processing of mourning aims to make the past part of the present reality through a return, this time symbolically and dialogically, to the memory of trauma.[34] Those who experience trauma are caught in a repetition compulsion that seeks to restore their capacity to feel anxiety and lack but in a symbolic, controlled reality, thereby reconstituting their disintegrated personality. I consider Dinur's choice to revisit the sites of trauma by means of writing fiction as an indication of his need to process mourning in a controlled context. Dinur detached himself from the concrete threat of direct confrontation with reality of the kind he experienced during the Eichmann trial, opting instead for a secondary, fictive reality. The novel *House of Dolls* does not feature a first-person narrator, and the characters are fictive and not directly related to the author. Dinur's own voice becomes manifest in a reality he, as an author, can control. It may well be the one domain in which he is capable of speaking up, with the laws of aesthetics protecting the witness, a safety net against collapse. Here chaos can be represented in language, which relies on the rules of logic and style, all of which shield against terror. Ka-Tzetnik expropriates the scream even from himself. He achieves this by means of mechanisms of displacement, where rather than Yehiel Dinur, it is millions of others who cry out his scream. The scream is of fictional heroes, written by a fictitious author. It is the exclusion that allows the scream to exist.

Yehiel Dinur took five names over the course of time. On his birth certificate, dated 1909, he appears as Yehiel Feiner. In Auschwitz, his name was converted into a number: 135633. After liberation, he immigrated to Palestine, at which point his name was Karl Zetinski. He continued using this name until his marriage, when he finally took the name Yehiel Dinur.[35] The word *dinur* is Aramaic for "from fire," and it appears in the Old Testament, in the Book of Daniel (9, 10), in Midrash, Talmud, and in the Kabbalist literature. Bartov explains it refers to a river of fire in the upper reaches of hell, pouring onto the evil dead to purify them.[36]

In all of his writings after the Holocaust, Dinur used the pen name Ka-Tzetnik.[37] In the novel *Salamandra*, it is Harry Preleshnik who represents Dinur and conveys his testimony. Though Ka-Tzetnik uses the third person in telling about himself, he clarifies that the story is based on true facts.

Dinur explained that some of his names were imposed by circumstances, while others were artistic choices. Until the Eichmann trial, he had been careful not to reveal that he was behind the Ka-Tzetnik pseudonym. Yechiel Szeintuch, Dinur's biographer, reported that in conversation, Dinur denied being the author of *Piepel:* "No, no. It wasn't me who wrote that. It was Ka-Tzetnik who wrote it, and I am not Ka-Tzetnik."[38]

In his final book, *The Code*, in which he did use the first-person singular, Dinur recounts how when the judges at the Eichmann trial put an end to the distinction between Ka-Tzetnik and Dinur, he felt so threatened that he passed out. About the reason why, as a writer, he felt the need to hide behind a fictive name, he wrote:

> It's such a simple and banal question, but once it passes from my ears to my brain there's an explosion. They are about to join the two identities into one and I will have to publicly attest to it. So, I escape from both into a no-man's-land, like a 'vegetable' in hospital.[39]

For Dinur, this plurality of names and their split use between fiction and reality served as a defense which he therefore could not give up. Asked to connect these diverse names, he collapsed in the courtroom together with his text.

The urge, as one who found himself in the pit of hell and was subsequently saved, to bear witness on behalf of those who did not return, was irrepressible. Ka-Tzetnik describes his mission in apocalyptic, visionary terms, and by introducing the myth of the salamander, as in his first novel.[40] This mythic animal is resistant to fire, and when a human being covers him- or herself in its blood, they cannot be harmed by the flames either. In Ka-Tzetnik's book, the salamander transforms into a metaphor for, or even symbol of, the writer's omnipotence.[41] For the only animal-in-the-flames has the words to describe, as he said, what happened in the ovens.[42]

The fire motif illustrates the clashing tendencies in Ka-Tzetnik's post-Auschwitz writing. On the one hand, writing as a calling and mission represents an impulse countering erasure: The salamander, who stands for Ka-Tzetnik, faces the all-consuming fire and is invulnerable to it. It can escape the inferno and assume the mission of the witness of the annihilating fire. In doing so, the salamander fulfills its commitment to those who also saw but did not return. On the other hand, we cannot completely ignore Dinur's morbid tendency to burn and be burned, over and over again, as if fulfilling the aggressor's aim to destroy him. This is what he writes when, in *Salamander*, the protagonist Harry Preleshnik enters the concentration camp.[43] Ka-Tzetnik renders the destructive powers inside him which are also expressed in his actual life.

Miron described in his article, "From Book to Ashes" how one day Dinur walked into the reading room of [Israel's] National Library in Jerusalem and requested access to a rare copy of his own first publication, hiding the small booklet and sneaking it out of the library. Coming back home, he set fire to what he assumed was the one surviving copy of the book.[44] Miron argues that it was not because he thought his poems were immature. Dinur's case, for Miron, mainly illustrates the dangers of violence turning against the self because of his survivor's guilt.[45]

Much research has been dedicated to the documentary aspect of Ka-Tzetnik's work.[46] Still, his oeuvre constitutes an exceptional representation of the personal and literary encounter of an authentic, primary, and naïve perspective with extreme trauma. In this chapter, I will be discussing Ka-Tzetnik's choice of poetic strategy: an envelope protecting the writer's mind against collapse. I will be looking at representations of screaming with reference to stylistic tendencies (kitsch) that undermine them. I will be showing that the textual practices representing the shout or howl render a kind of psychic processing in both protagonists and author. It is the role of this processing to protect and insert a barrier against the traumatic reality, a negative sublime that resists containment.

The novel *House of Dolls*,[47] on which my discussion focuses, contains materials which have so far escaped thorough examination. Its explicit description, straight from within the eye of the storm, deserves consideration. Ka-Tzetnik's words come from within the conflagration, and it is from that place that his howl emanates. What is the nature of his outcry? How is it represented? What are the psychological and the aesthetic mechanisms generating this representation, and how do they affect the reader? These are the questions that underlie the present chapter.

The Scream in the Poetic Text – Features

A scream expresses a personal voice with suddenness and force; it tends to be fragmentary and uncircumscribed and originates in distress and sharp pain. Each line in *House of Dolls* holds the sound of a scream. This will here be examined in terms of the four principles mentioned in the previous chapter: quantity (amplification or reduction); distinctiveness (sharpness or vagueness); coherence (fusion or splitting); and finally: value attribution (hierarchy or equivalation). The principle of quantity will be considered in terms of the volume of speakers' voices; distinctiveness will be examined with reference to the use of oppositions; coherence is tapped through the manner in which elements are fused into a whole; value attribution, finally, is studied by looking at the hierarchical relations in the conflictual form of the classical narrative. My textual analysis aims to show how these elements serve the book's kitschy style, a means the author uses to stave off collapse into chaos or muteness.

I will start off by presenting a characterization of the scream in terms of its *representation in language*, giving special attention to the element of amplification. Next, I proceed to the *formal level*, identifying two main narratives: a journey narrative and an apocalyptic narrative. As the novel unfolds, the latter takes over: it is with the apocalyptic narrative that the novel concludes. This leads me to a discussion of *kitsch as a defense mechanism*. A plurality of opposites and contradictions has a blurring but also unifying effect that comes to simulate an ecstatic bacchanal.

The Principle of Amplification

Ka-Tzetnik's writing amplifies a fundamentally grave reality by means of repetition and hyperbole. Repetition has a powerful effect of congestion and excess, prompting irrational feelings in the reader. This congestive and totalizing quality of the text is exemplified in the following quotations from the book:

Repetition (Multiple Anaphora):

The stillness exploded like a paper bag: *Shrieked* the barbed wires and *shrieked* the eyes strung out on them; *shrieked* the high heavens and *shrieked* the block rooftops.

(p.205)

No one knows from where the large vans bring the piles of clothing to the shoe factory warehouses day after day. *No one* knows where the people are who wore these piles of clothes, and *no one* pursues this thought to its logical conclusion: Where were these people taken to naked, unclothed?

(p.2)

Exaggeration or Hyperbole:

Harry stands amid hordes of bristling slaughter knives. *Everything* is red, crimson red. Around him, at him, myriad heads of drunken train conductors guffaw through gaping maws.

(p.18)

… *always*, before Harry comes, she has a *thousand* things to tell him. But the moment she sees him, she suddenly seems to *lose her tongue.*

(p.40)

> *Everybody* watched him with admiration and she would be so proud of him. She used to wish that winter would last *forever*, that it should *never never end* and that Harry should be home, *always*.
>
> (p.42)

> There wasn't *a word* in the world that could solace him and her; *a word* that would make up for the wetness of his coat, the fields hell soon have to slosh through.
>
> (p.45)

> … *countless* locomotives… leering faces… smokestacks… Daniella looks. Her brain swims. *Everything doubles. More. More. Tenfold, hundredfold, thousandfold.* They're *all* chasing her. In a minute they'll grab hold of her.
>
> (p.121)

Tautology:

> God! How casually Zalke stated: Nothing new in Kongressia ghetto. *The living aren't dead; the dead aren't alive.*
>
> (p.13)

Excessive Use of Punctuation

Intense, unrestrained emotionality is signaled by the pronounced use of punctuation like dashes between words, or question marks (often accompanying rhetorical questions), exclamation marks, and ellipsis (three dots). The following passage illustrates this style:

> Where are they being taken? How many more times will they be taken like this? Where's the van heading for now? Can this really be the last time they're being taken? At every roundup in the ghetto, he would think: This is the last time!… When he was deported from the ghetto, he was sure: This must be the last time!… When the "Lame Slave dealer" picked him out of the ranks at Camp Sakrau he knew that this must be the last time! Where's he being taken now? How many such "last times" are there?
>
> (p.227)

Intense Figuration

Ka-Tzetnik uses a great deal of metaphor. One especially prevalent metaphor derives from the semantic domain of volcanic activity. This metaphoricity maps the cosmic dimensions of a powerful natural phenomenon onto the Holocaust experience.

The Volcanic Metaphor

> There are moments when the pile of worn clothing in the center of the rag room bestirs itself suddenly like a *volcano* and sends a pervasive fear throughout the large room.
>
> (pp.1–2)

The novel in fact concludes with the volcanic metaphor:

> The pupils of his eyes flared up like *two seething volcanoes*, and the pain *erupted and streamed* into his every bone.
>
> (p.239)

The Full Container/Empty Container Metaphor

> Comes an Aktion and the German reaches into the ghetto as into a seed *bag* and *pulls out* a fistful; every seed that slips between the fingers gets a bit of a reprieve inside the gloomy sack....
>
> (p.13)

> ... Ardent wishes teeming in the human heart are like seeds ejected into the invisible womb of the cosmos.
>
> (p.23)

The container metaphor is especially prominent in descriptions of conditions of fullness/emptiness: Meeting Harry in the ghetto, Daniella "feels like a *bottle filled* to the cork *full*, but looking *empty*" (p.40 emphasis added – RD), and here is a description of the Muselmanns: "They moved through the camp [...] Like *hollow* men; *Empty* containers bobbing at sea" (p.91).

When the ritual of killing has been concluded, the chairs, now empty, at the center of the terrain are described as follows: "drained as *bottles* on a table after a sumptuous feast" (p.206).

Uses of Lack or Absence: Darkness (Absence of Light) and Silence (Absence of Sound)

Shadows emerge from courtyards, and when they enter the hall, their shadiness blends with the deep obscurity of the house. Amplification takes the form of an intensification of the color black; black shadows are swallowed by the blackness of the dark:

> The corridor leaving the house was already filled with human *Shadows* [...] Daniella turned up [...] as soon as she enters the *dark* corridor, she senses that its walls are already draped with *human shadows*, mutely waiting to dash out under the lifting curfew. [...] You don't see anymore, just as you *don't see a shadow* melting into a *dark corner*.
>
> (p.25)

Further emotional intensification is achieved by an anthropomorphism of the feeling of sadness:

> In the evening, at five o'clock, *grief is again locked up* in the houses. Glum and morbid, *it crawls* down the cramped walls, *bends over* the person and *reaches* the cup of sorrow to his lips.
>
> (p.27)

These quotes illustrate the intensity of the narrator's voice – it is a scream that penetrates the text's various layers. Perhaps, if this writing would only have aimed to constitute a loud outcry, it would have collapsed, much like Ka-Tzetnik's text collapsed in court. We must assume, hence, that the text includes a mechanism that protects it and that the scream's invasiveness is countered by a variety of other devices that shield against collapse. I claim that this defense mechanism takes the form of kitsch, a form which, while on the one hand being responsible for reiteration and amplification, also contains and enables the howl to be represented. I elaborate on this below.

The Principle of Distinctiveness: Dichotomizing Contours

Violent reality enters the protagonists' inner life suddenly, causing their world to split asunder. In the novel, this split is felt through dichotomization: An idyllic world is invaded by the powers of evil. Conflict, in Ka-Tzetnik's work, is always between polar opposites, dichotomies lacking subtlety and complexity. The reader is presented this dichotomous world in coarse and concrete, clashing terms.

The Representation of the Trauma Inherent in Opposition

Good Dream vs Bad Dream

The Good Dream: In Chapter 2 of the novel, Daniella reconstructs the night before the great journey and recounts how, too excited to fall asleep, she found herself leafing through her diary, where she read the following:

> Schoolboys and schoolgirls, now on their summer vacation, take frequent walks in the city park. Some lean over the wooden bridge on the lake and toss bits of bread to the *snow-white swan* gliding across the mirror of water like a *serene princess ensconced in reverie*. From the expression on her face, you can tell she regards herself *queen* of this realm: the park and all of us standing around *belong to her*. The sky and sun are her companions; the stars, her playmates. […] she goes sailing *majestically* back across her mirror-lake- a proud pauper.
>
> (p.17)

This text is written by an adolescent girl on the eve of the war. It offers a simple illustration of how Daniella's internal-phantasmatic reality is projectively reflected in the image of the swan. The image reveals a narcissistic, omnipotent world-view, in which Daniella – the swan – is at the center of the world. Such is her attractive power that it does not only dominate the above-mentioned others but also affects nature itself – sky, sun, moon, and stars. She rules them all. The Biblical allusion to the dream of Joseph reinforces this effect.

> **The Bad Dream, or Nightmare:**
>
> (...) out of the darkness of the park the white swan floats toward her. The long moonbeam streaming through the window flares into a lake. *The swan twins itself.* A brace of swans float near along wooden bridge. Daniella stands on an unknown shore. The lake is a *maelstrom of red and black.* Behind her back, countless trains prance and reel. The train engines have faces, like leering drunkards. They grind screeching slaughter knives into rails. Daniella wants to flee. She wants to save herself. But she can't. As if she were running against a gale. Her feet lift heavily, as though running under water. [...] The brace of swans suddenly spread white wings, beckon her to come to them: they will give her shelter. Daniella runs. The way is long. The nearer she gets, the further they recede. She stumbles. She is about to fall. She struggles frantically to reach them. She screams. But the scream sticks in her throat. Suddenly she feels herself plunging off a great height into a bottomless void, falling... falling.
>
> (p.18)

The good dream, placed to contrast with the nightmare, is one of many instances where Ka-Tzetnik uses opposition in order to create a one-dimensional, dichotomizing look at an extremely complicated phenomenon. In the face of disintegration and constant attempts at eradication, Ka-Tzetnik holds out two split positions: the ideal, perfect past, in which the narcissistic figure rules the world, on the one hand, and the cruel present, in which she transforms into a hounded victim in a threatening and perplexing reality.

The Principle of Consolidation: Convergence and Fusion

In the face of an extreme reality, Ka-Tzetnik looks for solutions that allow him to contain and represent it. Even though this reality drives him to dichotomize – split between past and present; victims and perpetrators – he cannot dwell with this splitting and is compelled to return to convergence and to fuse the extremes. His protagonists, who tend to be narcissistic in relation to themselves and symbiotic with others, are unable to tolerate separation and disintegration. In response they produce a loud clamor in which the fragmented reality comes back together again, undoing all possible differentiation. Consolidation into one loud scream is achieved by means of an ecstatic melancholic withdrawal and morbid incorporation of the void in the form of suicide or madness.

What the different types of screams in this novel have in common is the principle of convergence and fusion. The language reflects this in, for instance, an extraordinary amount of conjunction achieved by hyphenation – whether appropriately or not. Metaphor moves along a number of coordinates, all serving the principle of fusion, conjunction, and totality. First and foremost is the metaphor of water. Water is literally and associatively related to weeping and tears, but here water metaphorically covers everything, so all oppositions crumble and blend into one amorphous entity.

Even though Ka-Tzetnik uses metaphor and imagery in the fusion category, these figures of language act like metamorphosis rather than metaphor. Whether deployed as metaphor or as metonymy, figurative language is usually considered a transposition from one domain of meaning to another. This process, starting on the level of the concrete, involves abstraction. In the case of metaphor, transformation is linguistic and conceptual, the movement being from concrete to abstract. In Ka-Tzetnik's writing, a phrase like "a wave of clothes," is not merely a metaphor. It constitutes a singular, concrete metamorphosis unfolding right before our eyes. Metamorphosis means change of shape: we observe one object transforming into another. In the metamorphosis at hand, this transformation is from the domain of clothing to that of water (a wave) and it is a physical, real process. Where there is metamorphosis, the difference between literal and figurative is no longer relevant.

The crushed and broken image of the world is presented by a metamorphic mind that has become lost to itself (Harry's) – or by one which has chosen to die (Daniella's). Below I offer some illustrations of this morbid metamorphosis.

Expressions of Confusion or Mix-Up

In the novel's final description of Harry's madness, all distinctions vanish and everything blends:

> Everything swarms, wriggles [...] Everything is normal here. The wildest absurdity the soberest reality. Anything goes here, anything is possible, the way anything goes and is possible in insanity. Death and life dwell together here. Blood and wine are drunk from the same flasks. The Carrion Shed and the SS rooms are one. *Borders erased. Boundaries lost….*
>
> (p.234)

At the novel's end, when Daniella commits suicide, colors bleed into each other: "All around red… crimson red… a maelstrom of black and red" (p.241).

Uses of Metaphors as Metamorphosis

Volcano and water metaphors, like the metaphor of the shipwreck, fish metaphor, wave metaphor, water as a metaphor for purifying death, all of these function like metamorphosis to represent hermetically enduring, monolithic reality of mortal terror: "The ghetto atmosphere rushed in through the walls of the fortress called shoe shop like the sea into a floundering vessel" (p.56); "The whole ghetto is like a burning ship far at sea" (p.71); "[…] Hayim-Idl's plot suddenly seemed like a lone piece of wreckage on a sea of floating icebergs" (p.107); "Off in the distance, from among the *waves* of heads, the basket full of shoe lasts whited back at her like the mast of a *sinking sailboat*" (p.121); "[…] There, on the slide, her soul quivers like a *fish on the hook*" (p.208); "The doctor's mouth is like the *mouth of a fish*. Its corners arch all the way down" (p.211); "He felt as if he were *drifting through waves* of murk. His strength is leaving him and the shore moves further and further away" (p.226) "*Waves upon waves*, the walls of the stairs vestibule toss on a high sea. Yellow. Red. Waves toss him between open doors, and the swastika on Siegfried's belt buckle looms up *between the waves*" (p.237); "*The water will enfold her*. The *water* will rinse her body and *purify* it. The water will rinse her eyes and quench the fire raging in her head. She will lie deep, deep on the bottom of the lake, the way she's lying here, on the bed, only there it will be peaceful, soft, and free. The *lake water won't stop streaming* over her naked body and will cleanse it inside and out. She'll be pure, light, free" (emphasis added, p.188).

These two key metaphors, of the volcano and of water, map the existential condition of the story's main figures by means of semantic fields relating to uni-directional processes of disintegration, leading to a metamorphosis into ongoing total destruction, chaos, and indistinctness, where everything transmutes into everything.

Whereas metaphor is inherently figurative, not signifying actual change, metamorphosis tends to denote literal transformation.

Oxymoron, or the Fusing of Opposites

At especially ecstatic moments, the text becomes oxymoronic: "(…) now the marketplace was full, suddenly it was empty – at once full and empty" (p.11); "Daniella is sitting on her bed. Her head is full and empty" (p.82); "It was as in a dream. A static, immobile dream filled with emptiness" (p.232); "It's a bacchanalia of sound which is ear-splitting stillness, weeping which is laughter" (p.234).

Sudden disruption, on the one hand, and the rapid re-joining of the fragments in moments of ecstasy, on the other, reflect an ecstatic mental state characterized by the refusal to dwell in a traumatic reality. The novel generally is marked by a dynamic from flawless perfection, through a shattered reality, and into a unified reality in which the reunited parts are assumed into a chilling negative sublime, a homogenous reality of destruction and chaos: "As if lava has begun seething within the clothes heap and is about to burst out and swamp everything, everyone" (p.12).

The Principle of Equivalence: Collapse into Fusion of Opposing Narratives

Hayden White,[48] the philosopher and historian, has argued that in documenting a historical narrative we tend to impose patterns that produce coherence and meaning-giving hierarchies. He distinguished four types of historiographies: annals, chronicles, narratives, and philosophy.

Where historiography took the form of annal writing (referring to the Latin *annus* – year; hence, the term yearbook) traumatic events threatening human life, like death, destruction, famine, and flood, were registered as they unfolded over time. These were extreme events, selected for recording because of their important role in the struggle for survival. Annals tend to be written on scrolls and appear in two columns: one details the dates, the other the events. They represent real-life occurrences. There are no gaps in chronology, and no causation is provided. What ties the events together is chronology only. In this sense, the events are equivalent: there is no focus or center to organize and structure the events. Time in this type of text is referential and emerges in the act of documenting. No closure retrospectively structures the events, and there is no narrating voice. This choice to stick to chronology and abstain from an organizing, narratively meaningful idea, White argues, reflects an avoidance of moral positioning and meaning vis a vis the recorded events. Annals only record ongoing occurrences – they don't tell a story. They aim for objective historic documentation.[49]

In the genre of the chronicle, by contrast, while preserving chronology, the narrator's presence increases. Chronicles include a central subject, augmenting narrativity and adding coherent organization to the materials. The narrator of the chronicle is both present and conscious, maintaining a distance from his or her own expressions.[50] These two modes of writing are both guided by a principle of continuity. White discusses the world view of historiographers who observe this principle. He believes it reflects a deterministic approach in which humans are moved to action by events rather than assuming a position vis a vis them.

It is with narrative writing that writers' commitment to correspondence between the reality and time-bound order of events and the order in which they are recounted and documented ends. Narrative requires the emergence of causality and coherence as a type of relation that yields patterns. Closure is integral to this form, and through it the author expresses a moral stance in relation to the events.

While the philosophical text constitutes a kind of meta-narrative, attempting to present major, extremely generalized developments without reference to historic reality (one example is Hegel's model of thesis, antithesis, and synthesis, or the Marxist model), the life story (which is a personal history) dedicated to trauma deals with a complex encounter between actual experience during an extreme event and its reproduction and representation in language. Referring to White's approach to historic documentation, the question arises of what textual form would most appropriately convey traumatic events. Traumatic experience subverts one's experience of time, creating a rupture in the individual's personal history and familiar structure. As a result, the individual fails to fit the experience into her or his life's narrative. What will be the right story for this traumatic experience? Will the story about the trauma reorganize events in a coherent and hierarchical manner so that the narrative can offer new meaning, or will it rather resemble annals and chronicles in offering a mere timeline, without beginning, middle, or end? Alternatively – will the trauma narrative take a fragmentary, broken form whose constituent units are equivalent and lack coherence? Is this to be the form the authentic representation of trauma takes?

Ka-Tzetnik, in *House of Dolls*, chose a schematic, unifying type of narrativity that aims for closure, in spite of statements by both narrator and characters about their fragmented mental and existential state. The novel's major narrative form is that of the journey, but efforts to stick to this structure are undermined by another, competing narrative: one characterized by a belief in apocalyptic fate. Still, these two narratives jointly reflect a huge need for ready-made schemata telling chaos from culture and offering shelter from the turmoil that led to trauma. The obsession for structure, in this sense, testifies to a type of acting out that refuses to confront rupture, splitting, and fragmentation. Towards the end of the novel, nevertheless, the apocalyptic narrative takes over from that of the journey. In so far as the latter totally vanishes, the novel reasserts its drive to unity and totality, this time total negativity: the negative sublime.

The Journey Narrative

The novel *House of Dolls* proceeds along the classic structure of the journey narrative – a type of narrative that includes a beginning, middle, and end. Its organizing frame consists of a school trip planned to start some days before the new school year, in August 1939. The excursion, eagerly anticipated by Daniella, a young girl, for whom this will be the first time she travels without her family, ends with her suicide in a forced labor camp three years later.

The formal device of the journey reveals how external reality violently invades Daniella's adolescent world. I will closely consider this narrative sequence with reference to three central scenes: setting off on the trip, Daniella's removal from the ghetto to the labor camp, and, finally, her move to the 'House of Dolls.' Each ingression of violent reality, in each scene, further unsettles the protagonist's inner world. In the first scene, the threatening external world exists but is being denied; the external world invades in the course of the second scene, moving, however, in parallel with inner experience, which counters the threatening reality, removing it from consciousness by means of positive recollections. Realities, in the third scene, become muddled as the female protagonist is swallowed by the chaotic, senseless reality. The narrative structure proceeds towards the end's absolute closure: the act of suicide.

The relations between the narrative units are cumulative and hierarchical, with each event containing the main reason for the next. In this manner the narrative units proceed from a state of perfect order to one of chaos and brutal disorder among the powers of destruction, leading to the morbid conclusion. Below I illustrate the narrative structure's dynamic.

The Scene of Daniella's First School Trip

This scene is depicted with as many as possible idyllic features (a happy, united family, youthful mirth, an open and promising future). Soon enough, though, this turns into an ideal past, now crushed and broken. In spite of the presence of ominous elements (Daniella's nightmare-hallucination about the swans on the eve of the excursion and mention of the powerful military presence at the train station, for instance), these do not contrive to spoil the harmony of the life that is about to be shattered. Daniella's recollection of setting out on this trip will crumble in a cruel future, yet it will often return to her, at crucial points on her journey, in flashes and broken images.

The scene opens with a description of Daniella's excited anticipation of the trip:

> She, the fourteen-year-old schoolgirl, could not fall asleep that night before her first excursion. [...] Tomorrow, first thing in the morning, she is leaving for Cracow.
>
> (p.15)

When her father worries that this might not be the right time to set out on a school trip, with war about to break out, she dismisses his concern with adolescent nonchalance:

> What has a war to do with a school excursion to Mickiewicz's tomb in the Vavel? Today is August 27, and on September 3, when the new school year begins, the class will already be back. So, what's there to be afraid of? [...] how does all that concern her?
>
> (p.15)

She is very much looking forward: "What an adventure, what a cultural experience it's going to be! With her own eyes she will see her beloved Mickiewicz, almost all of whose poems she can recite by heart" (p.19). On the eve of the excursion, she packs the diary her older brother, Harry, gave her. She hopes to meet up with him during the trip. At daybreak, the next morning, she and the other girls march in an orderly row, while relatives, looking on from their windows, bid them farewell. Daniella's father and Moni, her younger brother, say goodbye at the train station, her father handing her the locket she forgot at home. It was his gift to her for her thirteenth birthday: its two tiny golden frames hold two pictures, one of her parents and one of herself and Moni. This farewell scene between Daniella and her father and brother is a classical specimen of kitsch:

> Daniella's head immediately appeared in one of the open car windows. The sky danced in the blueness of her eyes, and a sunny comb of breeze swept gaily through her golden tresses.
>
> (p.21)

The scene of course also includes the waving of a white kerchief and the vanishing view of the train:

> Daniella's eyes were riveted on her father: one hand waved a white kerchief high above his head, the other held on to Moni. The train moved gradually off. A gray emptiness unfurled rapidly between the endless ribs of railroad track. Daniella stood watching a long while, and her eyes cached the scene away forever.
>
> (p.21)

The Scene of Departure from Ghetto to Labor Camp – Parallel Realities

The next appearance of the narrative of travel is when Daniella has to leave the ghetto after being captured during the "girls Aktion." The train journey into an unknown future arouses her curiosity:

> Outside, a black ghetto night received them [...] An odd fear mingled with curiosity seized Daniella [...] An echo of something was playing back in her heart... something familiar... something she had felt before... the time she was getting ready for the first excursion in her life...Where is that school excursion now taking her?
>
> (p.84)

This excitement comes with reflection: Is it the death drive and an understanding that she is being taken to her death that causes this unusual state of mind? The landscape on the way, too, reflects this foreboding:

> The night winds itself about them and leads them off to the mysterious unknown. The blue-white caps on the militiamen's heads phosphoresce in the distance, under the yellow searchlight beams, like the eye whites of capering demons at the head of a mute night procession.
>
> (p.86)

The following morning the girls leave the "Dulag" (short for *Durchgangslager*, German for transit camp), about which the narrator has this to say: "The Dulag is the last stopover between the ghetto and mysterious death" (p.88). The girls pass through a street full of people who are being marched off to the train. Passersby are walking along both sides of the street and some of them stop to observe – mostly with indifference – the spectacle. Daniella is reminded of another procession, the time of marching with her classmates through the streets of Kongressia when heads of parents, mothers, and sisters were waving "pleasant trip" (p.120).

The contrast between the onlookers in the earlier scene and the impervious crowd leads the narrator to feel that the world goes on its way, but Jewish girls like cargo wait to be loaded up (p.123).

Both realities – the external reality in which Daniella is taken to the labor camp and the internal one, the recollected school excursion – unfold, for now, side by side, in parallel. Daniella hovers between hallucination and reality (p.123).

This stage of train travel is marked by awareness of an ambiguous world, with distinct facets – yesterday's idyllic world and the present, traumatic experience – even though both scenes feature train travel. The imagination produces a bridge which is likened to a silvery spider's web spanning between the two realities. This metaphoric bridge constitutes a kind of solution on the unconscious, hallucinatory level, allowing one to ignore the present by connecting to, and being nourished by, the past. This is why illusion is described as being so precious.

As Daniella muses on that idyllic trip, the reader learns, for the first time in the novel, of its traumatic conclusion, with the train coming to a halt and the girls being scattered and caught up in the massacre in Yablova market place:

> The first-term girls scattered in all directions and lost track of each other. Miss Helen didn't stop shouting: 'Girls, keep together! Remember, together!' Until she didn't hear her voice any more. The voice was lost somewhere in the frantic mob together with Miss Helen.
>
> (pp.123–124)

The Scene in the Dolls House – Mixed Realities

In contrast with the previous scene, dominated by the excursion, which preserved the distinction between inner and outer realities, with only an imaginary bridge linking them, now Daniella sinks into a chaotic reality. Shreds of images from different times and places add up to a cannibalistic reality dominated by "the wild echoes of a cannibal chant" (p.186). Daniella's crushed inner world is presented as she undergoes the traumatic experience of providing forced sexual services to German soldiers. The text does not directly render the cruel scene of the external reality: instead, we witness Daniella's torn inner perception, invaded and penetrated by external reality. In this reality, things have lost their distinct outlines.

She fantasizes killing the German soldier as he rapes her. This apocalyptic experience is underscored by the rhetorical device of synesthesia, the fusion of senses (voice and vision) and associations – both visual and narrative:

> But she feels the gong knells are looking in at her through the block window together with the German voices. They guffaw... the girls' heads spin before her eyes like wheels... wheels of a night trolley down Kongressia's drowsing streets... wheels of locomotives... WHEELS AWAY TO VICTORY!... Jeering faces of conductors... She is in her room... and now she is in Metropoli station among the girls of the transport... [...] Knives cut the wheels - she will grab a knife and slash the German's body when he's lying on her. [...] Night. Crimson night.
>
> [...] She stabs and slashes with the knife, and the blue inscription FELDHURE is red, flooded with German blood. [...] The block fills with Germans. Uproar. Commotion. Countless black boots. A seething caldron. German. Shouts. Guffaws. No more bars. No cages. Everything unloosed, No wheels.
>
> (p.185)

In this nightmarish reality the following three features stand out: shattered boundaries, total confusion of reality components, and infinite dimensions. All boundaries are gone. Past and present, the heads of girls and train wheels, screams and laughter – it all bleeds together into one boundless, ecstatic reality.

The Competing Apocalyptic Narrative: The Nightmare

The novel starts off with a familiar literary form, the journey narrative, in which the protagonist encounters a variety of situations that are occasions for growth and maturation. But by the end of the novel when Daniella faces death, she seems to have remained the same 14-year-old girl, pure and innocent as she was at the start. She remains an eternal adolescent. Her mode of mental coping, it could be said, takes the form of the entrenchment of a pattern manifest from the very beginning of the novel: in spite of its ostensibly evolving structure, it is a chronicle with a foretold end.

The many types of texts dedicated to the Holocaust often mention the discrepancy between victims' intellectual and conceptual equipment and the atrocities they had to confront. Reality always is a step beyond one's conceptual frame of reference, which therefore falls short and does not allow either to understand, let alone predict, the phenomenon in question. Ka-Tzetnik's protagonists know something about what is to come due to their active imagination and a sense of foreknowledge. Daniella's awareness of her fate is communicated right from the start of the novel on the eve of the war. This is not about rational knowledge. And nor does it have mystical, metaphysical origins. What she knows stems from her inner world which takes visual and narrative form as the novel moves along. What it represents lacks external criteria – a narcissistic perspective, whose core image is that of the swans in the "bad dream."

This nightmare gains explicit, literal importance as the novel unfolds. In this its role is not unlike that of the oracle in Greek myth. Yet in contrast with Greek tragedy, which is all about the hero's struggle against fate, Daniella's nightmare does not change: its meaning only intensifies as reality bears it out.

The nightmare includes three notable features: massive and exponential growth of threatening objects; unclear validity of the dream world, and a powerful disorientation in time. All this goes into producing an experience of totality; the emotional component is stretched to its limits. When the girls are "loaded" onto the train, Daniella is, once more, accosted by this nightmare:

> … *countless* locomotives… leering faces… smokestacks … Daniella looks. Daniella looks. Her brain swims. *Everything doubles. More. More. Tenfold, hundredfold, thousandfold.* They're all chasing her. In a minute they'll grab hold of her. She trembles. *She's seen all this before!* Exactly, exactly the same, the same locomotives, the same leering faces, the same chilling fear. *Everything, everything the same!* But she doesn't know *whether she saw it then in reality* and is now *having a nightmare, or whether that was the nightmare. Who so wise as to fathom the cryptic writing an unseen hand will from time to time draw on the panels of our dreams?*
>
> (p.121; emphasis added – RD)

Once she arrives in the forced labor camp, she is pursued by the sounds of the gongs, which remind her of the clangor of the trolley at night.

This actual manifestation of fate's writing produces a sense of timelessness, undoing the structure of the travel narrative.

In the scene describing the medical exam, reality unfolds exactly as in the internally produced nightmare's writing. The metaphoric bridge between then and now in earlier hallucinations now transforms into the real material of an intolerable reality: the bridge, which the Nazi sentry paces. Later on from this bridge she will be shot dead by the sentry. In the scene of the girls' medical exam, Daniella, waiting in line for her turn, looks through the window and this is what she sees:

> The SS sentry on the bridge leans over the wooden railing, tosses bits of bread to the two white swans gliding across the lake. The line moves closer to the table. The girls' naked arms are like long necks of white swans [...] The kalefactresses put a new girl at the table. The two gliding swans are framed in the KB window, float in a pair across the gloss of lake. Behind them the bridge... the bridge! the same bridge!... - she is on an unknown lake shore. The swan twins. *A brace of swans float toward her*. [...] She's being chased. The swans spread white wings. She runs toward them... Two kalefactresses seize her by the arms: The girl ahead of her at the table is almost done.
>
> (p.210)

Soon after the examination, as Daniella finds out her life is saved, for the time being, the swans vanish and the lake is empty (p.212).

Daniella kills herself in the novel's final scene. The swans, which in the writing of fate deliver her verdict, freeze, "like two marble statues in reverie [...] gaze at her... call her" (p.241). Daniella, moving away from her friend Fella, walks toward her death. Now she enacts her nightmare, which appeared "on the panels of our dreams" (p.121) – as the narrator put it. Here, Daniella enacts her death wish, which the novel already held out like a prophecy at its beginning. In this reality, both time and movement freeze. The two swans majestically represent death by first having become petrified and next, following the fatal gun volley, by moving off again, away from the camp, carrying Daniella's life on their wings into eternal goodness.

This undermining of one narrative by the other mainly has the effect of amplifying the powerfully obsessive dependence on a schematic structure which presumably will frame and order a reality that cannot be contained.

Trauma imposes a broken representation of experience by means of a fragmented rhetoric. But, unable to contain rupture, Ka-Tzetnik makes a huge effort to create both structure and style, countering this fragmentation. The novel's structure which split into two opposing narratives, eventually comes together again in an apocalyptic, all-consuming narrative. This leaves us with one ecstatic narrative, that of the negative sublime.

Kitsch as Literary Style: Poetic Defense Mechanism

Paradoxically, it was Ka-Tzetnik's need to frame and represent trauma, that led him to adopt kitsch as a style. While a literary text including an overflow of emotions can be considered sentimental,[51] it is when sentimentality goes hand in hand with worn-out, overly familiar imagery and immediately recognizable clichés, that it deserves to be called kitsch. One illustration is the sunset at the end of the massacre on the Yablova market square:

> The setting sun reddened the water and it looked like jets of blood spurting heavenward from Yablova market. Then the sun went down. The sky shaded itself with a strip of black night so it could afterwards claim it had not seen what took place in Yablova market.
>
> (p.125)

Other illustrations involve a volcanic metaphor: "As if lava has begun seething within the clothes heap" (p.12) or an apocalyptic image: "Harry stands amid hordes of bristling knives. Everything is red, crimson red. Around him, at him, myriad heads of drunken train conductors' guffaw through gaping maws" (p.18). The same goes for the scene of Daniella's murder-suicide:

> From out the *darkness* Daniella's *white*-draped figure moved off. She was pacing straight for the lake, moving into *the reddish* light of the wide camp road. The night crouching on both sides of the barbed wire opened *red*, inflamed eyes and tensely followed the movements of the delicate form of the girl in the *white* linen nightgown coming directly into its waiting maw. [...] The *twin swan statue* suddenly came to life. The gunburst had frightened them out of their marble serenity, and with outspread wings they went gliding quickly away from the camp shore, as if bearing on their *white* wings the tortured life of Daniella Preleshnik.
>
> (pp.242–243)

While trauma is defined as a breakdown of conventional concepts, Ka-Tzetnik opts for kitsch – a style that typically confirms the indisputable. Ka-Tzetnik is serious about kitsch, not ironical, grotesque, or reflective. Below I will look into this puzzling poetic choice, but first, I will discuss the concept itself.

Kulka[52] describes kitsch as involving a choice of objects or themes with a ready-made powerful emotional charge[53]; these objects and themes are immediately and effortlessly recognizable; moreover, kitsch does not add to or enrich our associations regarding them. Though it is emotionally intense kitsch lacks reflective qualities. The relentless stream of words, rhythms and images has a congestive effect and produces a sense of flooding, triggering sensational experiences that captivate readers. It is kitsch's emotional charge rather than any literary merit that guarantees its success.[54] Kitsch does not risk an avant-garde or unconventional approach: with its simple language and extreme transparency, it needs no interpretation. Kitsch always goes for the broadest possible common denominator and is entirely transparent: nothing is left to the imagination.[55] Anchored in stereotype, depicting subject matter in a conventional, formulaic manner, kitsch shuns the new and singular.[56] Rather than offering aid in cultivating our sensibilities or sharpening our perceptions, it tends to cover over true emotions.[57]

Milan Kundera, in his novel *The Unbearable Lightness of Being*,[58] defines kitsch as a style that seeks to confirm what already exists. The emotions it evokes must be of a kind that the masses can share. Thus, kitsch is rooted in conventional ideas and recognizable images, its true function being to serve as a barrier keeping death and confusion out of sight.[59] Kitsch captures readers' attention, seducing them with its stereotypic, clichéd structure which contributes nothing new. Simultaneously, it blunts readers' perception, keeping them captivated in a form of hermetic enchantment. Kitsch's self-deceptive aesthetic is an escapist genre frequently used for commercial advertising or propaganda, aiming for maximum, undemanding exposure. Seeking to offer instant satisfaction, it resonates the most undemanding, superficial aesthetic.[60] Omer Bartov, in his article "Kitsch and Sadism," has drawn attention to the glaring discrepancy between Ka-Tzetnik's charged subject matter and his literary choices – which Bartov argues result in "juvenile literature."[61]

In *Kitsch and Death*,[62] Saul Friedländer, discussing kitsch in the context of Nazi ideology, asserts that kitsch and death remain incompatible.[63] Kitsch relies on an overload symbol, a ritualistic-ceremonial atmosphere around death, and dread.[64] Friedländer believes the combination of kitsch and death results in a literary style reflecting negative transcendence: a blind destiny which leads to inevitable destruction.[65] This blend of kitsch and death does not aim to arouse tragic horror. It looks at death in a ritualistic manner: stylized, "beautiful death" replete with aestheticized atrocity, glorified terror wrapped in an ecstatic honey trap.

By definition, kitsch addresses extreme situations with an inappropriate effort to cover up. Trauma is a breakdown, forcing people to deal with a reality that diverges from or exceeds their conceptual framework. This requires repositioning themselves vis a vis reality. Ka-Tzetnik however opted to describe extreme situations in a style whose main feature, as we have seen, is reiteration and confirmation of things as they are.

Using kitsch, Ka-Tzetnik can dwell on the description of atrocities, wallow in apocalyptic scenes, wrapping them in an excess of words and imagery which eventually, and paradoxically, transform into a screen that hides the source of terror. Kitsch, in this sense, is a poetic defense mechanism that produces an envelope of aestheticized horror. This evident fascination and delight in apocalypse suggest the Lacanian concept of *jouissance*.

In contrast with Freud's pleasure principle which seeks for the release of tension and homeostasis, *jouissance* is beyond the pleasure principle in so far as it orients itself to the Real.[66] *Jouissance* is the excess feeling which does not achieve satisfaction because there is always an unrepresentable excess.[67] Freud argues that the pleasure principle functions to take emotional charge to a state of equilibrium: by means of release and drop in emotional charge emotional intensity is moderated. The pleasure principle, in other words, regulates emotion and restores homeostasis. Lacan's *jouissance* by contrast is an emotionality that exceeds pleasure: it is addictive and excessive and when fully brought to bear it leads to death. Discussing *jouissance*, Lacan also refers to the symptom – the latter always causes distress and hence prompts removal. The symptom however is persistent and will not let the subject get rid of it. The *jouissance* produced by the insistent symptom also causes pain. Yet it is the painful symptom's continued grip on the subject that prevents processing and locks the subject into endless melancholy.[68]

A Crack in the Inner World: Two Types of Acting – Out

The nightmarish reality Ka-Tzetnik screens by adopting kitsch stands revealed in two contradictory symptoms, namely, two types of acting-out. On the one hand, a dichotomous, polar universe divided into good and evil, black and white, life and death – supported by a distinctly stable, unambiguous and totalizing base; on the other, an unraveled reality, where boundaries are breached, and everything leaches into everything, a chaotic fusion that takes the form of a rampant confusion between victims and perpetrators. These two types of acting-out serve as a defense system that keeps chaotic reality separate from the egregious anxiety it produces.

In *House of Dolls* the characters experience a deep inner split. The broken realities, in this writing, are always treated as dichotomous and clashing. Things break abruptly, the moment is unannounced. The word "suddenly" fills the text, and comes to show the acute nature of the change that traumatized people undergo:

> A shudder *suddenly* ran through him when he placed his other hand on the stack [...]. [...] Passing the doorway of the rag room, the pile of old clothes insinuates itself into the corner of his eye. *All at once* it seems as though people like himself are lying there [...] There is no more strength for wanting. *Suddenly* his hand starts trembling. He wants to reach out, hold on to something, save himself. [...] *All at once* his feet tear away from the spot [...].
>
> (pp.60–61)

The suddenness of trauma, its rupture, confronts people with an alien reality. In the novel it is Daniella and Harry who experience fracture, and subsequent splitting, most keenly: "Her own life now lay at the foot of the heap of old jackets and trousers [...] *Two existences. Severed and sundered. No connection or bridge between them. Which is reality and which nightmare?*" (p.10; emphasis added – RD). When, at the end of the novel, Harry opens his eyes after passing out during the Nazis' cannibalistic rampage, he notices the camp commander standing right by his side, and:

> He lay as if bound to a *sacrificial altar*. He raised his eyelids, looked upward, saw as through a fine-spun veil: now everything is transparent, now it's all blurred. Now he sees, hears, understands and knows everything that happened to him, and now he knows nothing at all. [...] *Beside him on the floor lies his life like an infant of his*. Any moment now the black boot will crush it, and it won't show any more from under the boot sole. Any second now. *The infant lies beside him....*
>
> (p.236)

Ideal Past vs Traumatic Present

Splitting has the effect of arousing a powerful melancholy of the kind typical of rupture that can be neither healed nor processed. This breach portrays the past as idyllic and perfect, and it vies with a cruel, intolerable present. Ka-Tzetnik's work, in this sense, presents us with the melancholy of nostalgia: the past seems better than it was, and cannot be set aside. Daniella, more than any of the other characters in the novel, is given to this constant yearning for the past in view of the difficult present. On the eve of the war, the world, in her eyes, is totally good: "A bright world, radiant as an early-spring morning. A world full of mystic lures that beckon to young hearts. Summer's end, 1939" (p.15). From the here and now, the past appears as "A beautiful dream gone, forgotten. But it still ripples through her being, softly, tenderly, like the lingering, dying whisper of a harp-string; like the haunting echo of a melody of yearning. A melody of another world –" (pp.13–14).

We get to know very little about Daniella's close family. By means of the tiny photographs – one of her parents, and the other of Daniella and her youngest brother – in the locket she gets just before setting out on the fateful excursion we glean something of an ideal image of the Preleshnik family. Here Daniella appears

> In her school uniform, two blond, white-ribboned braids tumbling down to her breast. Beside her, on a round straw table, sits three-year-old Moni, in a white sailor suit, his velvet eyes rounded at the queer black picture box in front of him.
>
> (p.20)

Elsewhere in the novel, we gain some idea about the past through another look at these pictures. It is a precious, intimate moment during Daniella and Harry's last encounter in the ghetto:

> Harry took the locket in his hand, turned it over. There, his father's face looked up at him with deep blue eyes, the very eyes he and Daniella inherited from him, and by his father's head, the gentle face of his mother, the face he loved and worshiped above all in the world. 'The loveliest couple in the world, Pa and Ma,' she whispered.
>
> (pp.49–50)

All we learn about the family is through their reflection in these photographs. What we see is a middle class, bourgeois family, harmonious and pleasant, whose banality confirms the regular order of things. These images, which for Daniella evoke an ideal past, are standard images characteristic of their place and time. Very many families were immortalized in the same manner: posing similarly against the same background. From the perspective of kitsch, the idyllic past of these moments becomes a banal, conventional representation, with a touch of self-deception. But when such a representation appears in the context of a dichotomizing confrontation with a cruel, hyper-real present, the resulting impression is shocking. In this sense the melancholia represented through the irreparable breach perpetuates a type of mourning in which the depressed self is locked into a compulsive repetition of identification with the lost object.

Symbiosis – Fusion with Chaos

House of Dolls, then, laments a lost, idyllic past from the perspective of a broken world; the novel deals with this loss by means of acting it out through either madness or death. Both solutions reject the possibility of acknowledging fracture: they do not tolerate dwelling on and accepting states of fragmentation. While insanity ecstatically reaches for wholeness, contact with death cancels the forces of life. Both are driven by a fundamental need to repair what's broken through contact with something lost that was unbroken in the past. One illustration of this type of denial of fragmentation or boundaries is in novel's description of Daniella and Harry's symbiotic relations. The developmental stage of these protagonists' symbiotic self-other relations, goes hand in hand with the principle of fusion. They have not matured into autonomous, separate, and distinct personalities. Refusing to acknowledge that their reality has crumbled, they cannot make it cohere rationally with the idyllic reality they have spun.

Daniella and Harry: Symbiotic Self-Other Relations

At the forefront of the novel is the relationship between Daniella and Harry. They are siblings in a symbiotic relationship, which, in the course of the novel, fails to pass through separation and differentiation. Right from the start, an incestuous element is suggested, mainly through the motif of twinhood. The characters are described as resembling each other, both physically and in their ways of expressing themselves.

Physical Similarity

Here is a reference to the siblings' physical resemblance:

> Not just the eyes; all of Daniella's face now evoked Harry: the same chiseled mouth, the same twin white rows of teeth, the identical shadow between the lower lip and chin.
>
> (p.77)

Figurative Similarity

This type of similarity is reflected in the siblings' shared metaphoric of trees, land, and water. These metaphors are so conventional that one feels that each character in the novel could have used them. Still – they are in fact used only by Daniella and Harry.

Metaphor Likening Tree to Man

Both siblings use the tree as a metaphor describing their condition in the world. When he is alone in the sick room, Harry climbs on a chair to look out, from a high, barred window. From there he observes a sapling, onto which he then proceeds, romantically, to project the full charge of his emotions:

> Whenever he looks at this tender *tree* a gnawing sadness grips him, often so oppressive that he can't breathe. He forgets he is himself a prisoner here. It hurts him to see the wall looming over the tender sapling with its hideous back, blocking it off from the world.
>
> (p.101)

During her stay at the "Dulag," from which she will be transported to the forced labor camp, Daniella sees that the wall and ceiling bear engravings. Seeking for a sign from Harry, her eye falls on this:

> On the ceiling above her is a symmetrical, skillfully drawn tombstone. In the center of the tombstone is a Star of David with *a tree* beside it. The top of the *tree* lops down, snapped at the trunk. Beneath the *tree* a column of names [...] Maybe she'll find some sign of Harry here too!
>
> (p.113)

Both brother and sister use projection by way of expressing their wishes and their "self."

Mother Earth Metaphor

Describing beautiful days in the ghetto, Harry refers to the earth as feminine, a mother:

> The black, *soft-pleated earth, the warm earth, soaked into its bosom* the brow's sweat together with ghetto tears. The sky stretched free and boundless overhead.
>
> (p.106; emphasis added – RD)

Daniella, in the train taking her to the forced labor camp, sees the passing scenery as follows: "Far off, a sun-congested sky bent over the *earth like a mother* offering the bare fullness of her breast to the mouth of her suckling" (p.123).

Water Metaphor

Towards the end of the novel, brother and sister both use a water metaphor to express distress. The act of immersion in water evokes, via ritual acts (like Christian baptism), states of dissolution and chaos.[69] But while ritual actually removes the subject from their condition through reconstitution and reconfirmation of their identity, Daniella and Harry remain stuck in this metaphoric state. The following is for instance about Harry: "It was as in a dream. He heard the voice as through thick walls, as with clogged ears, as though he were under water" (p.230). And in the case of Daniella: "Everything is happening as under water. [...] The whole thing happened as in a vacuum" (p.201). Here, the two can be seen to enact a metaphor already suggested in the nightmare, right at the beginning of the novel: "Daniella wants to flee. [...] Her feet lift heavily, as though running under water" (p.18).

Similar Perceptions of Reality

Daniella and Harry share a perception of reality as indistinct from nightmare. The following is about Daniella:

> Her life lies at the foot of the heap of old clothes, [...] *Two existences*. Severed and sundered. No connection or bridge between them. Which is reality and which nightmare? [...] Can she be living these two separate lives simultaneously?
>
> (p.10)

And this is about Harry:

> He was lying on the floor by the stairs and he felt that his life now lay on the floor beside him like severed object [...] He lay as if bound to a sacrificial altar [...] Is his life still alive, or has it already been crushed? He is right here, and he isn't here.
>
> (p.236)

Conceptual Similarities

The major similarity between these two characters is in the conceptual domain, and it is reflected in the narratives that guide their lives: that of divine chosenness and that of divine sacrifice.

The Narrative of Divine Chosenness

From the very beginning, Daniella's diary writing is presented as something special. The diary is not a mere chronology, the personal jottings of an adolescent girl: it reveals a talent for writing for which she also gains a prize. The diary entries themselves, too, reflect powerful self-worth, as I have already mentioned, a narcissistic self-sense represented in the description of the swan on the lake (p.17). Daniella observes Vevke looking for her before the transport, and this touches her. She felt a moment of chosenness which engulfs her, and this feeling seems to distill her pain (p.117).

Harry's chosenness is mentioned against the background of the forced labor camp itself. Of all the inmates, he is selected to be the camp doctor. Why is not clear to him. Of all the people in the camp. It must be fate that he had been chosen to stay alive in the camp (pp.92–94). This chosenness of his is not merely observed among his fellow prisoners; Yaga, the German woman, too perceives it while seeing Christ in him (p.109).

The Narrative of Sacrifice

The two sexual scenes in the book occur in the context of the bacchanalian excesses of a party, whose main motif is human sacrifice. The following description is of Daniella:

> Daniella's ears are clogged. The bawdy German shouts reach into her ears as from a great distance, like the wild echoes of a cannibal chant. [...] She lies bound as in the cage, knees astraddle, unable to move a limb.
>
> (p.186)

And this is about Harry, after the wanton celebration in the German quarters: "He was lying on the floor by the stairs, [...] He lay as if bound to a sacrificial altar" (p.236).

These descriptions of the protagonists in the context of the ritualistic, sexual actions of a cannibalistic society that practices human sacrifice, reveals the text's hidden mythic image. This image fashions the characters as sacrifices made to pagan gods, serving as the perpetrators' scapegoats and outcasts. These two scenes describing ritual blend in order to express an impulsive eruption of acting-out in the epic encounter between life and death, between instinctual passion and sacrificial acts.

Identical Motif of the Color White

One type of poetic trace that reveals the text's unconscious is the motif of whiteness, which equally marks and traverses both Daniella's and Harry's consciousness. In the case of Harry, white attaches to the principles of life and death, while in Daniella's white is associated only with death. This, for instance, is how the sick bay of which Harry is in charge, is described: "The only bed in the room was a crib. The Commander had picked it up some place because it was *white*" (p.91). This bed has no function. Sick people are not allowed to be put there: When Harry reaches the sick bay after loading the corpses onto a van, he casts a look into the room and his eye is caught by how

> The *white* sheet was spread on the *white*-lacquered crib taut, smooth, without the slightest wrinkle. Not a prisoner has ever lain on this bed. The *whiteness* of the sheet splashed against his eyes like a *white* puddle; a blood puddle not red but *white*.
>
> (p.225)

Here the text ties Harry's looking at the white sheet to the puddle of blood, associated with Daniella, at the end of the novel. The image of the white puddle imposes itself on Harry, and, crazed, he gazes at it: "On the site of the bed there was now just a blob of *white*. The blob floated around the sick bay, swelled and burst, its *white* shreds hanging down from the dark corners" (p.225; emphasis added – RD). Dragged to the Germans' quarters, he notices "A window set with panes – faces of daylight. A *white-lacquered* sill" (p.230; emphasis added – RD). Later on, in a state which might be either dream or reality, he lies on the *white*-lacquered bed, the forbidden baby's crib, and all he begs for with a howling plea- is a tear.

The white crib stands in a sick bay where people only come to die. At the end of the novel Harry is put on this crib, leading to an experience that more than hints at a wish for life, which will, eventually, be fulfilled.

While at the end of the novel, as far as Harry is concerned, the color white – here in the form of a crib – still connotes life, in the context of Daniella, white, though infused with glory, is only associated with expressions of her death wish. And though black and white both dominate the background, white eventually dominates: "red verged on black, the brace of swans stood *white*, like two marble statues in reverie" (p.241). Close to death, in a trance, Daniella has a vision of Harry who "stands in a *white* smock as shrouded in cloud" (p.241).

From early on in the novel, Harry always appears in Daniella's dreams with a reference to the color white: "The image of Harry swathed in *white* floated up before her eyes. What is this thing which keeps coming up in her dreams? What does it signify?" (p.70). Towards the novel's end, Daniella looks out over the scenery, the white swans call out to her: "the brace of swans *whiten* like twin statues against the dark of night, gaze at her… call her…" (p.241). When she dies, Daniella is described in terms of her white nightdress: "From out the darkness Daniella's *white*-draped figure moved off" (p.242). The two white swans mirror her: "swans stood *white*, like two marble statues" (p.241). Unable to watch Daniella die, "Fella couldn't bear any more to look into the night, at the splotch *whiting* on the road" (p.244). The white stain that crazed Harry's mind is now mirrored in the white stain representing Daniella in this chapter. This composition in white comes to an end with Fella, left behind with the locket, looking at Daniella's image:

> With both hands she held the locket up to her eyes. Out of the photo Daniella gazed at her, dressed in her *white* sailor-collared school outfit, two thick *white*-ribboned braids tumbling down to her breast, her gaze serene, pure, innocent.
>
> (p.244)

White here serves to symbolize both Daniella's death drive, as well as the purity and innocence of one whose life was tragically and cruelly cut short. Physically speaking, white is composed of all other colors. Homogenization, non-differentiation, or non-distinction is a central force of the death drive. In that sense the color white is metaphysically appropriate. The choice of white as the color representing

Daniella's suicide suggests a homogenous solution in the face of a reality that is far from homogenous and which the protagonist grows unable to contain. The solution held out by the conclusion of this novel is in the spirit of what Freud called the death drive.

The portrayed physical, mental, and emotional similarity between the two key characters, Daniella and Harry, gradually melds them into one character. The novel's amplification of the morbid scream is personified by a ghost-like girl from Oswiecim, who keeps appearing and vanishing mysteriously throughout the narrative. She represents the essence of the howl, a poetic expression of the unspeakable, the traumatic core.

The Girl from Oswiecim: Making Trauma Present

The girl from Oswiecim fled the town after the Nazis erected the annihilation camp Auschwitz on its premises:

> She's about fourteen or fifteen years old. Maybe much older, or maybe much younger. It's hard to say. *Sometimes she looks like a child, sometimes like an old woman.* No telling when and how her face will next transmute right before your eyes. [...] *She never says a word,* and her eyes are always downcast. [...] There hasn't been an Aktion in the ghetto that *she hasn't foresensed* [...] She always vanishes before an Aktion and [...] furtively steals back in when the trouble is over. *With the same instinct by which a jungle beast senses* the enemy's approach from miles away, she always *seems to scent* the Germans in advance. Not a single Jew in Oswiencim [sic – RD] was saved. Not one of her family survived. *No one knows what her eyes beheld there. She simply slipped in here one midnight with the dilapidated man's shoe in her hand. What secret does this man's shoe contain that the girl hugs it so to her heart?*
>
> (p.35)

The girl from Oswiecim first enters the narrative during a chaotic scene in the ghetto: There's a big outcry in Hayim-Idl's room when the girl attempts to grab back a used man's shoe from little Bella who's been playing with it innocently. The ecstatic peak of this scene is reached when Hayim-Idl's cries out: "Piss on the free world! The devil take a free world that asks for the blood of my Bella!" (p.34). The little girl only stops wailing after the shoe passes on to Hayim-Idl. We get to know very little about the girl from Oswiecim in this scene whose name is not disclosed till the end of the novel.

The father's outburst stirs up an intense emotional, irrational reaction, suggesting traces of unconscious materials. Rather than representing a realistic life, the figure of the girl from Oswiecim has a narrative core that conveys something fundamental about trauma. With a covert maneuver, a *mise en abyme*, reduplicating the core narrative, the girl from Oswiecim becomes the mysterious center of *House of Dolls*. The girl suffers from mutism and harbors a terrible, unutterable secret.

Only a metonymic remainder is left to point at the trauma: a used man's shoe which she absolutely refuses to part with. In the shoe, a real object is re-presented, an object that survived the traumatic event. It also stands, metonymically, for a world that was destroyed. This is not a random choice: for Ka-Tzetnik the shoe invokes the person who was supposed to be wearing it. It evokes the living person's ability to move from one place to another, but also the absence of the dead person, when all that remains is the useless shoe. The shoe thus serves as a kind of bridge between what in Lacanian terms would be called the Real – the inaccessible domain of trauma – and the symbolic domain which is subject to representation.[70]

As mentioned, another conspicuous feature of the girl from Oswiecim is her mutism, which is her sole testimony to the victims who did not survive. Lyotard, referring to the victims' muteness, introduces the concept of the *differend*[71] to describe a situation in which both addresser and addressee –without whom there is no testimony – have become neutralized. Something seeks expression but fails as a result of severe, unrepresentable transgression. The girl's muteness and the shoe to which she clings are gestures or traces of trauma which cannot otherwise find expression.

The girl from Oswiecim is depicted as an animal in the forest: unconscious, she uses her instincts and senses – the sense of smell, which is considered particularly primitive – to survive. In psychological terms she manifests a profound, primitive level of traumatization. Freud argued[72] that the first shock of trauma is experienced unconsciously, as something that occurs outside conscious time and space. From this perspective, the girl stands for trauma frozen in its most primitive state. Injury, in this state, is suspended, animalistic, instinctual and unconscious. External reality has violently penetrated the self's vulnerable inner world. Ka-Tzetnik uses the girl from Oswiecim to zoom into this primitive state of traumatization: he successfully conveys her core experience, with its silent horror. This is how he evokes the unconscious trauma in the here and now, presenting it in the form of a wordless acting out.

Only once more does the girl from Oswiecim make an appearance in the novel, and here too her appearance is conveyed through unconscious material, in Daniella's dream about Harry (pp.65–69). Now alone in the ghetto (Harry having been put on transport to Auschwitz), Daniella dreams she is working together with him in the ghetto's sewing workshop, showing him how to unfix things. She hallucinates her powerful longing for Harry and her dread of never seeing him again. In her dream, Harry pulls a parcel out of his pocket and in it is the girl from Oswiecim's used man's shoe. Daniella wonders whether

> [...] it was the same shoe or its mate which Harry had brought along with him escaping from Auschwitz. Harry clutched the toe of the shoe with both hands and ripped the upper off the sole. Suddenly it looked as though he were holding open the *jaws of a crocodile*. The two rows of white wooden pegs *looked like jagged teeth in the crocodile's maw*.
>
> (p.66)

Schultze grabs hold of Harry and tells him: "From Auschwitz the shoe came and to Auschwitz it will return!" (p.66). When Daniella asks why he is provoking the Germans, Harry replies: "I'll go on tearing *the shoe's maw* or it will *swallow me alive*. Do you want it to *devour* me as it did Ferber? I won't let it. I'm stronger than they!" (p.66; emphasis added – RD). On waking from this dream: "when she sidled her eyes about the room, [Daniella] saw the Oswiencim [sic – RD] girl returning to her bed with the black man's shoe hugged to her heart" (p.69).

In part of the dream, the girl from Oswiecim does not appear: the shoe acts synecdochically, representing the lost one as well as the source of dread: Auschwitz. Harry holds the shoe and this symbolizes his fate. Daniella is only preoccupied by the question whether the shoe Harry has in his hand is the one the girl from Oswiecim had with her, or whether it was "its mate." But in any case, in the dream Harry's fate is sealed. Once the shoe is identified with terror itself, any context in which it appears is contaminated by this terror. In the dream, Harry struggles with the shoe which transforms into a crocodile. The comparison between the torn shoe and the crocodile's maw is based on physical similarity between an inanimate object and an animal. But this is not the only way the image steps up the terror. What resonates here are the great, archaic creation narratives. *Enuma Elis*, the Babylonian creation myth, describes a gigantic struggle between the archaic ocean, Tiamat, mother of all living things, and Marduk. While Tiamat seeks to preserve chaos, Marduk strives for order. In the struggle between these powers, Tiamat creates mythical crocodile-shaped monsters who threaten to devour anything within their reach.[73] Ka-Tzetnik's echoing of this mythological monster intensifies the horror. This is a question of survival: will the victim let himself be devoured or will he heroically struggle against his fate? The circle closes as Daniella's wakes and sees the actual girl from Oswiecim, holding the shoe. This is how Ka-Tzetnik brings to bear unconscious materials which are never articulated but intangibly inhere in the horror they cast and through the avoidance of contact with them.

The story of the girl from Oswiecim brings terror to the brink of consciousness. The girl herself remains mute and unconscious of herself: the reader learns about her only through her actions, e.g., in terms of acting-out. Terror is rhetorically amplified by inserting mythological echoes which reinforce the kitsch. The authentic traumatic core is wrapped with ready-made literary materials associated with terror. These produce emotional intensification to the point of ecstasy. This is the type of amplification that gives vent to a howl but gets in the way of processing. Excess, cliché and kitsch arguably do not only seek to step up emotion, they also, paradoxically, come to occlude it by way of a false envelope. This type of material signals the presence of the unconscious source which is behind the screen it constitutes, but leaves it as something that does not know itself.

World View: The Negative Sublime

For Ka-Tztetnik in *House of Dolls*, Auschwitz is another planet, mysterious and occult, whose main trait is its enormity: "The camp looked outlandishly vast, as if the whole world were contained within its confines" (p.135). He attempts to render the experience of an unfathomable negative sublime. Still, I have been able to identify no more than two sentences in the entire novel referring to the insufficiency of either language or the imagination in the face of that reality: "Hentschel swims day in, day out in a sea of blood, in an inferno of human misery *for which no language in the world has the idiom*" (p.150; emphasis added – RD).

The novel singularizes terror as something impenetrable, inexpressible. The strange tale about the van reminds of the story about the girl from Oswiecim:

> Where is the van taking the bones? At what kind of place will it pull in? Then where will they be taken from there, from that *mysterious* place? *Always* taken to a *mysterious* place, and *always* taken from that *mysterious* place to another *mysterious* place. *Always taken. Always* tossed into big, dark vans. *Always* bones stacked on bones. Sometimes live bones, sometimes dead bones. It's all the same.
>
> (p.227)

These expressions all suggest that the writer treats trauma as a negative sublime yielding an almost ecstatic experience of terror and pain: I have shown that Ka-tzetnik's main means of achieving this effect is by amplification through excess and repetition. Longinus, the 3rd-century Greek philosopher and rhetorician, mentioned amplification as a rhetorical principle used in the description of the sublime, but he drew a distinction between a sense of the sublime achieved through elevation, and one based on amplification, of elaboration that conveys abundance while "dwelling upon" the addressee.[74] Ka-Tzetnik uses much pictorial language, together with overelaboration and overstatement to elicit readers' feeling and shock. Longinus, already, is conscious of the pitfalls of excess and abundance in the representation of the sublime, which he believes may result in a false sublime: "It is true that it often needs the spur, but it is also true that it often needs the curb."[75] The representation of the sublime is ill served by flowery language, pathos, excess and childish simplicity – all meant to procure an effect in the listener rather than focusing on the greatness of the thing itself. The false sublime, Longines argued, might be only an "appearance of elevation which will rather be despised than admired."[76]

Rather than rendering Auschwitz as inscrutable and mysterious, another planet, which cannot be imagined or consciously evoked – as Ka-Tzetnik, among other things, describes it, the narrative he produces stands out for its kitsch. The use of familiar, banal material seems to serve to protect him and allow him to represent the negative sublime. The use of kitsch can be considered a compulsive repetition of the familiar in the face of the unfamiliar; a distraction enacted by a fugue into banal language and style. The rhetoric of kitsch generates an aesthetic artifice whereby the howl or scream, in the face of the negative sublime, is nevertheless expressed.

The Ritual of the Negative Sublime: Two-Fold Morbid Closure

One of the ways in which Ka-Tzetnik's novel articulates the negative sublime is by means of the absolute dichotomy between blameless victims and demonic perpetrators, with the triumph of the latter an end foretold. The victim in pagan rituals symbolized the outcast, thereby instituting the system's boundaries and order of signification.[77] The victim, in the present narrative, is innocent, and in this very position he or she negates the demonic system that puts them there.

The theme of Jewish innocence versus the Nazis' demonic evil takes many different forms throughout the novel. Daniella has a pure untainted soul and she sacrifices her own life to avoid pollution by German evil, forced upon her through cruel rape. The protagonist's young age, her blue eyes, the clash between her innocence and her terrible fate – all of these evoke the traditional life of the saint who sacrifices herself for the sake of ultimate purity. In contrast with the victims who, due to their self-sacrifice, will remain eternal adolescents, the Nazis are portrayed as primitive, evil participants in pagan cannibalistic rituals: "The bawdy German shouts reach into her ears as from a great distance, like the wild echoes of a cannibal chant" (p.186). We are thus offered a strictly dichotomous, quasi-religious worldview, dividing between superior and inferior beings. This cleansing is related to death and melancholy,[78] and to instinct beyond the pleasure principle,[79] which seeks to revert to a more primitive state (i.e., non-life). In his earlier mentioned book *Reflections of Nazism*, Saul Friedländer, discussing the association between purity, kitsch, and death, explains that purity is represented by a whole range of symbols like for instance protagonists' tender age, or their blue eyes.[80] In *House of Dolls*, the protagonist is an eternal adolescent who faces the powers of evil undaunted by the ultimate price of self-sacrifice.

House of Dolls' dominant principle of unity and fusion leads, however, to the depiction of a homogenous world, with evil taking over everything. Lacking an external point of reference, Ka-Tzetnik presents a chaotic, unbounded reality whose polar opposites collapse into one another, becoming inextricably fused. The result is withdrawal into a metamorphic world, through a pagan, ritualistic abandon to death. With all boundaries obliterated, chaos and irrationality rule everything. It is in this sense that the book's dominant perspective is that of the negative sublime.

The novel concludes with a two-fold ending: Chapter 18 is dedicated to the end of Harry's story, Chapter 19 to that of Daniella's. Even though Chapter 18 includes the final encounter between brother and sister, the novel does not end there. While Chapter 18 is recounted from Harry's perspective or close to it, Chapter 19 issues from the mind of Fella who witnesses Daniella's murder-suicide. Do the twin souls eventually become unified? Are they finally fused? Or do their differential reactions to trauma keep them distinct and separate?

Harry: Madness

Harry is mostly presented from Daniella's perspective, and often through her adoring eyes. But in Chapters 8, 11, and 18 we glimpse him without this prism. Here we witness an impulsive character with a "phantasmagoric dream" attitude to reality (p.91).

In the novel's final two chapters Ka-Tzetnik suggests a nightmarish reality: Partly, the narrative in both chapters unfolds simultaneously – as Harry, courtesy of madness, passes from life to death in order to be reborn as an infant, and Daniella sacrifices herself by committing suicide. Chapter 18, the penultimate chapter, strangely presents entry into the domain of death, on the one hand, through a bacchanalian touch achieved by hedonistic forces (represented by the erotic relationship with Yaga the German Nazi), and finally by reference to Daniella as a "doll," on the other. The struggle between death and life impulses culminates in madness, which intimates re-birth. Into all this come driving two vans, one of them conveying corpses from concentration camps, and the other Daniella and Yaga who are brought in to serve the Germans' debauchery. The death drive is represented metaphorically by the van carrying the dead bodies, while the life drive is conveyed in a perverse erotic ritual joined by both perpetrators and victims.

Death Wish: The Corpses Van

When Harry, needlessly, leaves the sick bay of which he is in charge, to see for himself how the corpses (among them his friend Zanvil Lubliner's) are being stacked onto the truck, he is ordered by the SS driver to do the job himself. Like Odysseus in the land of the dead, he climbs onto the truck, where in the dark the dead bodies, collected from other camps, appear as mysterious guests:

> Here, in the van parked on your own parade ground, they look like fantastic guests, like corpses of distinction. First, because they have been brought from the outside, from beyond the barbed wire, from a mysterious somewhere which you cannot plumb, though you know it exists, just as the inhabitants of one planet know of the existence of another planet, yet cannot visualize what it's like there.
>
> (p.218)

Death here is viewed with reference to alien planets (p.221). Inside the van the laws of reality change. Things grow indistinct getting in the way of order. The world in the van is chaotic, the "self," losing individual consciousness, drowns (p.224).

Back in the sick bay, Harry suffers from actual hallucinations and language becomes metaphoric:

> In the sick bay, on the table, *the necks of the empty bottles stood in three straight rows, one beside the other, mute and impassive.* Their muteness amplified the dull roar in his ears. *He could no longer bear the order, the compactness on the table.* [...] His brain was reeling. He felt as if lie were drifting through waves of murk. His strength is leaving him and the shore moves further and further away.

> [...] He's going under. The shoreline recedes, melts to a gray fog. [...] *He felt himself drifting under the murky waves.*
>
> (pp.225–226)

Harry loses touch with reality. The metaphor of death via the corpses-van stays formative of the morbid reality: "From the distance, day peered in through the block gate *as into the dark of a sealed van*" ([emphasis added], p.226).

Life Wish: The Ritual

We can make sense of the novel's closing events with reference to fantasy. Harry and Daniella meet at a Nazi sex party in the concentration camp. Daniella, who is forced to do sex work, arrives in the camp with German Yaga. Yaga persuades Siegfried, a German officer, to let Harry join an orgy at the Nazi quarters. She seduces Harry, calls him a saint, and drags him along to the party. Again, Harry feels he's crossing a line: his ride in the corpses van has removed the boundary between life and death, and now he joins the depraved Germans (p.230). Fantasy waxes and takes over. He is being dragged through the kitchen. Reality becomes more tenuous, transforming into a carnival, cacophonous and shocking, where sex and death blend and language turns into oxymoron:

> Hitler gapes down wild-eyed from the kitchen wall: What's a Jew doing in the German kitchen? Kill! Kill! Kill!... 'Oh, Holy One!' the drunken German woman whimpers. Drop dissolves in drop. *Infinity and split second, melt into one. Beginning and end converge. It's a mute life-and-death puppet show.*
>
> (p.232)

Looking at the drunken Nazi party from his place near the door, he feels: "as on the threshold between dreaming nightmare and waking to madness" (p.233). He is in a Nazi dungeon and not only hears, but even seems to see, the wild drunken voices. The disorder he was yearning for when in the sick bay now presents itself:

> Bottles empty, part empty, overturned and scattered rolling on the floor among wiggling naked bodies of men and women moaning and panting drunkenly [...] The wildest absurdity the soberest reality. Anything goes here, anything is possible, the way anything goes and is possible in insanity. Death and life dwell together here. Blood and wine are drunk from the same flasks [...] Borders erased. Boundaries lost. [...] It's a bacchanalia of sound which is ear-splitting stillness; weeping which is laughter. [...] Everything turns red.
>
> (pp.233–235)

This pagan scene includes sex, and blood and wine drunk from the same bottle. The fluids pour into the ecstasy of total transgression. One contribution to the morbid kitsch derives from the sexual excess following the pagan rite.

From this chaos, a naked, German woman emerges and approaches Harry. Drunkenly, she tries to put her arms around his legs and she gazes at him with her blue eyes. Harry thinks: "What are Daniella's blue eyes doing here? 'The loveliest couple in the world, Pa and Ma!' Dani's voice... The eyes scream... Her mouth gapes... It's Daniella's voice screaming to him. He hears. He clearly hears. 'HARRY! HARRY!!!'" (p.235) Then Harry faints. When he comes to, the camp commander stands near him:

> Stillness... Beside him on the floor lies his life like an infant of his. Any moment now the black boot will crush it [...] Any second now. The infant lies beside him....
>
> (p.236)

Harry is saved in a grandiose finale which has the effect of a *deus ex machina.* Once more he is dragged to his sick bay, all his phantasms mixed up:

> Turmoil. He must be out of his mind! But he did see and hear! But where did Dani come here from? But he plainly saw Daniella's eyes! He's out of his mind! But he did hear her cry: 'Harry!' The screams are still ringing in his ears. What happened to him next? Where is he now?
>
> (p.238)

Though he tries to reconstruct reality, each attempt leaves him in another version of the same nightmare. Did the corpses van really happen? Did he find himself in the Germans' quarters and was it Daniella he saw there?

At the end of the novel, Harry is psychotically flung between a wish to die and a wish to live, taking him eventually to a kind of rebirth. The ecstatic description of this rebirth seems to represent a sort of acting out, with protagonist blending into narrator, a type of fusion that covers up splitting and the fragmentation of the conscious experience. The pathetic turn to Hippocrates, pleading with him for tears, though testifying to deep distress, maintains the overwhelming ecstasy to the very end of the novel.

Daniella: Suicide

In *House of Dolls'* final scene, Daniella kills herself, but only after passing her diary and the locket she has kept with her throughout to Fella, asking her to pass them on to Harry. Fella senses that Daniella is about to end her life, but she has no way of stopping her. The figurative description of the camp suggests that the scene is set for Daniella's death:

> To the right, opposite the KB, the round lake lay on the ground like a head flung into the Joy Division, the wooden bridge like a noose around its neck. [...] Mid-lake, where red verged on black, the brace of swans stood white, like

> two marble statues in reverie, [...] the brace of swans whitens like twin statues against the dark of night, gaze at her... call her....
>
> (pp.240–241)

Daniella separates from Fella and walks towards her death. She now enacts the nightmare which was written on the "panels of our dreams" (p.121), as the narrator put it:

> From out the darkness Daniella's white-draped figure moved off. [...] Facing her are the brace of swans like a twin sculpture. The night answered the gunburst with wild, rollicking laughter. [...] The twin swan statue suddenly came to life. The gunburst had frightened them out of their marble serenity, and with outspread wings they went gliding quickly away from the camp shore, as if bearing on their white wings the tortured life of Daniella Preleshnik.
>
> (pp.242–243)

Daniella, in this scene, fulfils her death wish, an end foretold. Time and movement grind to a halt, something majestically represented by the two unmoving swans. They float away from the camp after the volley of shots, their wings carrying Daniella's life into everlasting peace.

Daniella dies unvanquished by an abject world. Her death-sacrifice underscores the cruelty and injustice of her fate. Her act of self-sacrifice at the end of the novel carries a religious aura, reinforcing the sublime aspect of evil. The morbid closure, including both madness and suicide, reflects a state of mind marked by profound and irreparable melancholy in the face of an unmanageable reality.

The symbiotic psychological relations between brother and sister, together with the novel's final ecstasies of madness and death, show acting-out at work as a coping mechanism which refuses to accept the traumatic experience of splitting and fragmentation: Ka-Tzetnik reaches for a lost whole, at the price of sanity and life.

Unresolved Contradictions in Ka-Tzetnik's Writing

Experienced as a "black hole," as a negative force, trauma has a strength and continuity beyond what the mind can grasp and/or conceptualize. In this sense we may call it a negative sublime, triggering feelings of cessation and nothingness, together with pain and existential terror. Trauma affects a person's deepest resources, touching on the most fundamental questions of being. Traumatic contents relate to destruction, annihilation, and loss, the nature of absence and nothingness.

Ka-Tzetnik's work is replete with unresolved contradictions. Biographically speaking there are hiatuses between the artist's statements and reality. On the one hand he commits himself to document reality objectively, to the point of self-erasure, turning his eyes into a camera that records reality mechanically and objectively, even after his death. He even promises that he will serve as a mouthpiece to those who perished, and he gives up his name for a generic pseudonym which means camp-inmate. On the other hand, however, Ka-Tzetnik's world is revealed as solipsistic and subjective offering no anchors to lean onto, beyond himself. When given the opportunity, in court, to fulfil his commitment, his text collapsed: Ka-Tzetnik fainted.

Still, he was the first Hebrew novelist to tear the veil of silence surrounding the Holocaust. This forced him to seek a representative response to a reality that had not been represented before. He chose literary fiction for his mode of testimony, and for the scream as a disintegrated mode of expression which at once lacked boundaries yet was forceful. His scream typically is rendered by a rhetoric of hysterical, obsessive amplification. It is an expansive mode of expression with excessive imagery, accompanied by visualizations that border on the pornographic aiming to arouse intense emotion. His rhetoric represents trauma in a mode of *jouissance* involving two kinds of acting out: one represents a split and dichotomous world of victims and perpetrators, or of an idyllic past versus a nightmarish present, while the other presents a world dominated by radical evil and devoured by boundless chaos. In such a reality, language loses its symbolizing power, presenting metamorphic states in which, everything is swallowed by everything before the reader's eyes, as a result of the author's ecstatic state of mind.

In the fictional space, Ka-Tzetnik does not collapse: he uses poetic defense mechanisms, and most prominently kitsch. This stylistic choice might appear surprising: Ka-Tzetnik represents the traumatic experience in a manner that seems to completely clash with the fragmented, torn and boundless nature of trauma, by opting for "the immoderate where moderation is needed."[81] Even though Ka-Tzetnik directed his gaze at the negative sublime, he chose to attach himself to a clichéd symbolic. This leads to a discrepancy between experience and its representation, revealing a false-looking negative sublime. Longinus mentioned the possibility of a false sublime where exaggeration was applied inordinately.[82] In Ka-Tzetnik's case we can observe the inordinate, though it takes an inverse form. An extreme phenomenon like the Holocaust requires rhetorical restraint rather than amplification.[83] The type of poetic restraint Ka-Tzetnik opts for in his writing, kitsch, undermines the effort to represent trauma in adequate dimensions. His stylistic choices display the kind of fascination and arousal he himself experienced as a writer. It is an emotional experience that may well trap readers in trauma and block their judgment. This fascination lures readers into a state of mind that mimics and reproduces the trauma, a second-order experience taking them, too, down into a paralyzing melancholy that prevents processing. The processing of trauma does not demand total emotional control, yet it resists full surrender to trauma's boundlessness. In this sense Ka-Tzetnik's text remains trapped within the defense mechanism of kitsch.

Yet, if we peel away the text's layers of symbolic, clichéd language, and focus on its acting-out rhetoric, it offers insight into the nature of trauma. In spite of the hysterical excess in the unprocessed, uncontained representation of the past, we may perceive how his style generates traces leading to the profoundest traumatic core. A case in point is the rhetorical strategy the author uses around the girl from Oswiecim. I believe this girl embodies the authentic, unspoken remainders of trauma: the dimension of Lyotard's *differend*, the negative sublime which takes the form of the traces of an inaccessible, ineffable yet authentic world.

Overall, this analysis shows how Ka-Tzetnik's work is dominated by unresolved contradictions, reflecting an unelaborated tension between the commitment to objective documentation of the Holocaust and his subjective, solipsistic perspective and poetic defense mechanisms, of which kitsch was the foremost. These contradictions reflect the broader challenges of representing and comprehending the Holocaust, a problematic that marked Ka-Tzetnik's entire literary legacy.

Notes

1 Ka-Tzetnik, *House of Dolls*, trans. Moshe M. Kohn (Simon and Schuster, [1953] 1955), 244.
2 Ka-Tzetnik, *House of Dolls*.
3 This is what Yehiel Dinur (Feiner) writes for the Israeli Army journal *Bamahaneh* in May 1961, following the first day of the Eichmann trial in Jerusalem; Yehiel Dinur, "I Accuse", *Bamahaneh*, May 1961. [Hebrew].
4 Parts of this chapter appeared in my doctoral dissertation, Rina Dudai, *Modes of Coping with Trauma in Holocaust Literature* (Hebrew University, 2000). [Hebrew], as well as in my article, Rina Dudai, "Kitsch and Trauma: A Reading of Ka-tzetnik's *House of Dolls*", *Mikan* (2006), 125–146. [Hebrew] and in Rina Dudai, "Pain and Pleasure in Poetic Representations of the Holocaust", in *Marking Evil, Holocaust Memory in the Global Age*, eds. Amos Goldberg and Haim Hazan (Berghahn, 2015), 233–265.
5 Dinur Yehiel, https://www.youtube.com/watch?v=m3-tXyYhd5U.
6 Tom Segev, *The Seventh Million: The Israelis and the Holocaust*, trans. Haim Watzman (Picador, 2000), 4. https://archive.org/details/seventhmillionis0000sege/page/4/mode/2up?q=salamandra&view=theater.
7 Dudai, *Modes of Coping*; See also Shoshana Felman, *The Juridical Unconscious* (Harvard UP, 2002); Amos Goldberg, *Trauma in First-Person: Diary Writing during the Holocaust* (Indiana University Press, 2017).
8 Dan Miron, "Between Book and Ashes", *Alpayim 10* (1995), 196–224. [Hebrew].
9 P. Azay, "The Man from Planet Auschwitz", *Haaretz*, 16 June 1961.
10 Omer Bartov, "Kitsch and Sadism in Ka-Tzetnik's Other Planet: Israeli Youth Imagine the Holocaust", *Jewish Social Studies 3:2* (1997), 42–76; Miron, "Between Book and Ashes".
11 Tom Segev, *The Seventh Million: The Israelis and the Holocaust*, trans. Haim Watzman (Picador, 2000), 4.
12 On the various versions of the manuscript and its translation, see Yehiel Sheintokh, *Innocent Speaker: Conversations with Yehiel Dinur* (Bet Lohamey Hageta'ot, Dov Sadan Institute, 2003), 261–306. [Hebrew].
13 Segev, *Seventh Million*. There are inconsistencies between the biographical details provided by Azay, Miron, and Segev respectively. They concern, for instance, Dinur's place of birth, Sosnowiec in Miron and Azay, but Katowiece in Segev. Further inconsistencies include the translation and publication of *Salamandra* and Dinur's date of birth (1909 vs 1917); cf Yehiel Sheintokh, *Salamandra: Myth and History* (Carmel, 2009), 31–34. [Hebrew].
14 Sheintokh, *Salamandra*, 34.
15 Segev, *Seventh Million*.
16 Miron, "Between Books and Ashes", 197.

17 A.B.T. "A Life That Is Death, and Death That Is Life", *Haoved Hatsioni*, 1 June 1953. [Hebrew].
18 A.B.T. "Life That Is Death".
19 Zvika Dror, "Nightmare Holds Him in Its Grip", *Massa Davar*, 20 April 1990. [Hebrew].
20 Aharon K. Bertini, *Gilyonot* Adar-Nisan (1953). [Hebrew].
21 Moshe Pelli, "The Art of Ka-Tzetnik's Type of Holocaust Literature", *Mahut 2* (1990), 148–159. [Hebrew].
22 Asher Nahor, "The House of Dolls", *Herut*, 6 March 1953. [Hebrew].
23 M. Halamish, "The Clock Overhead", *Al Hamishmar*, 20 January 1961. [Hebrew].
24 Talpaz, "Trilogy of Death", *Davar*, 11 August 1977. [Hebrew].
25 G. Shofman, "Salamandra", *Davar*, 20 December 1946. [Hebrew].
26 P. Lander, "The Girl from the House of Dolls", *Haaretz*, 16 October 1953. [Hebrew].
27 Yotam Reuveni, "Salamandra", *Ot*, 12 January 1972. [Hebrew].
28 Yeshurun Keshet, "Dolls House by Ka-Tzetnik", *Davar*, 27 February 1953. [Hebrew].
29 Mordechai Yaffe, "On 'House of Dolls'", *Al Hamishmar*, 6 June 1958. [Hebrew].
30 Emanuel Ben-Gurion, "House of Dolls", *Davar*, 12 April 1953. [Hebrew].
31 I will describe this process in detail below.
32 Bartov, "Kitsch and Sadism", 48–51.
33 Bartov, "Kitsch and Sadism", 51
34 Cathy Caruth, ed., *Trauma: Explorations in Memory* (Johns Hopkins UP, 1995); Dori Laub "Bearing Witness or the Vicissitudes of Listening", in *Testimony: Crises of Witnessing in Literature, Psychoanalysis, and History*, eds. Shoshana Felman and Dori Laub (Routledge, 1992), 57–74.
35 Sigmund Freud, "Beyond the Pleasure Principle", in *The Standard Edition of the Complete Psychological Works, Vol. 18.*, ed. and trans. James Strachey (Hogarth Press, 2001), 7–66; Eric L. Santner, "History beyond the Pleasure Principle: Some Thoughts on the Representation of Trauma", in *Probing the Limits of Representation: Nazism and the Final Solution*, ed. Saul Friedländer (Harvard University Press, 1992), 143–154.
36 Yechiel Sheintuch, *KATZETNIK 135633, Dialogues with Yechiel De-Nur*, ed. Carrie Friedman-Cohen (Ghetto Fighters' House & Dov Sadan Institute, 2003), 13–14. [Hebrew].
37 Bartov, "Kitsch and Sadism", 42–43.
38 See Sheintuch, *KATZETNIK*, 13–14.
39 Sheintuch, *KATZETNIK*, 28.
40 Ka-Tzetnik, *Ha'Tzofen* (Kibbutz Meuchad, [1987] 1991), 85. [Hebrew]; cited in Sheintuch, *Salamandra*, note 1, pp. 69, 71; also, in Sheintuch, *KATZETNIK* 135633, 13–14.
41 Sheintuch, *Salamandra*, 55.
42 Sheintuch, *Salamandra*, 55. On Ka-Tzetnik's sense of literary vocation, see also Sheintuch, *Salamandra*, 40–56.
43 On the mythological salamander see Sheintuch, *Salamandra*, 307–364, and especially pp. 312, 317, 319, 323.
44 From Galia Glasner-Heled, "Who Does Ka-Tzetnik Represent?" *Dapim 20* (2005), 190. [Hebrew] and Goldberg, *Trauma in First-Person*, 73; his argument is that Ka-Tzetnik's "rhetoric works on the same level as the murderer's sadism." See also, Dudai, *Modes of Coping with Trauma in Holocaust Literature* (2000), 106; Dudai, "Kitsch and Trauma", 135.
45 Miron, "Between Book and Ashes".
46 Miron, "Between Book and Ashes", 223.
47 See for instance Sheintuch, *KATZETNIK 135633*; Sheintuch, *Salamandra*; Iris Milner, "The Evil Spirits of the Shoah: Ka-Tzetnik's Literary Testimony to Death and Survival in the Concentrationary Universe", in *Holocaust History and the Reading of Ka-Tzetnik*, ed. Annette F. Timm (Bloomsbury, 2018), 67–78; Uri S. Cohen, "Ka-Tzetnik, Primo

Levi, and the Muslims", in *Holocaust History and the Reading of Ka-Tzetnik*, ed. Annette F. Timm (Bloomsbury, 2018), 153–166.
48 Ka-Tzetnik, *House of Dolls*.
49 Hayden White, "Historiography as Narration", in *Telling Facts: History and Narration in Psychoanalysis*, ed. Joseph Smith and Morris Humphrey (Johns Hopkins University Press, 1992), 284–299.
50 Hayden White, "The Value of Narrativity in the Representation of Reality", *Critical Inquiry 7:1* (1980), 15–16.
51 White, "Value of Narrativity", 17.
52 Abrams, *Glossary*.
53 Tomas Kulka, ed., *Kitsch and Art* (Penn State University Press, 1996), 95, 97.
54 Kulka, *Kitsch and Art*, 28.
55 Kulka, *Kitsch and Art*, 97.
56 Kulka, *Kitsch and Art*, 27.
57 Kulka, *Kitsch and Art*, 37.
58 Robert Nozick, "On Kitsch", in *Kitsch and Art*, ed. Kulka Tomas (Penn State University Press, 1996), 99.
59 Milan Kundera, *The Unbearable Lightness of Being*, trans. Michael Henry Heim (Harper Perennial, [1984] 2009).
60 Kundera, *Unbearable Lightness of Being*.
61 Matel Calinescu, *Faces of Modernity, Avant-Garde, Decadence, Kitsch* (Duke University Press, 1987).
62 Omer Bartov, "Kitsch and Sadism in Ka-Tzetnik's Other Planet: Israeli Youth Imagine the Holocaust", *Jewish Social Studies 3:2* (1997), 42–76.
63 Saul Friedländer, *Reflections of Nazism*, trans. Thomas Weyer (Harper & Row, [1982] 1984).
64 Friedländer, *Reflections of Nazism*, 22–23, 35.
65 Friedländer, *Reflections of Nazism*, 40.
66 Friedländer, *Reflections of Nazism*, 17.
67 Alain Vanier, *Lacan* (Other Press, 2000).
68 Dylan Evans, *An Introductory Dictionary of Lacanian Psychoanalysis* (Routledge, 1986), 91: "The pleasure principle functions as a limit to enjoyment. At the same time, the subject constantly attempts to go beyond the pleasure principle. However, the result of transgressing the pleasure principle is not mere pleasure, but pain, and this painful pleasure Lacan calls Jouissance: jouissance is suffering".
69 Jacques-Alain Miller, *Le partenaire-symptôme: l'orientation lacanienne, 1997–1998* (Martinière, 2003).
70 Itamar Grinwald, Adela Yarbro Collins, Margaret Mary Mitchell, and Hans-Dieter Betz, "Paul and Ritual Theory: The Case of 'The Lord's Supper' in 1 Corinthians 10 and 11", in *Antiquity and Humanity: Essays on Ancient Religion and Philosophy*, eds. Adela Yarbro Collins and Margaret Mary Mitchell (Mohr Siebeck, 2001), 159–187.
71 Jacques Lacan and Jeffrey Mehlman, "Seminar on the 'Purloined Letter'", *Yale French Studies 48* (1972), 39–72.
72 Jean-Francois Lyotard, "The Differend: Phrases in Dispute", trans. George Van Den Abbeele (University of Minnesota Press, [1983] 1988), 22–23.
73 Josef Breuer and Sigmund Freud, *Studies on Hysteria*, ed. and trans. James Strachey (Hogarth Press, 1955).
74 Wilfred G. Lambert and Simon B. Parker, *Enûma Eliš. The Babylonian Epic of Creation* (Oxford, 1966), Tab. 1: 134–145.
75 Longinus, *Longinus on the Sublime*, trans. W. Rhys Robert (Cambridge University Press, 1907), Chapter 12, 77. https://ia600204.us.archive.org/12/items/LonginusOnTheSublimeTheGreekTextEditedAfterTheParisManuscriptWith/longinus_sublime_Roberts.pdf.

76 Longinus, *Longinus on the Sublime*, 45, Chapter 2.
77 Longinus, *Longinus on the Sublime*, 55, Chapter 7.
78 Julia Kristeva, *Powers of Horror: An Essay on Abjection*, trans. Leon Roudiez (Columbia University Press, 1982).
79 Sigmund Freud, "Mourning and Melancholia", in *The Standard Edition of the Complete Psychological Works, Vol. 14: On the History of the Psycho-Analytic Movement, Papers on Metapsychology and Other Works*, ed. and trans. James Strachey (Hogarth Press, 2001), 243–258.
80 On the death drive in Freud, see Freud, "Beyond the Pleasure Principle".
81 Friedländer, *Reflections of Nazism*, 28.
82 Kulka, *Kitsch and Art*, 44.
83 Longinus, *Longinus on the Sublime*, 68.

References

Abrams, M. H. A. *Glossary of Literary Terms*, Thomson Wadsworth, 1980, 283

A.B.T. "A Life That Is Death, and Death That Is Life", *Haoved Hatsioni*, 1 June 1953. [Hebrew].

Azay, P. "The Man from Planet Auschwitz", *Haaretz*, 16 June 1961.

Bartov, Omer, "Kitsch and Sadism in Ka-Tzetnik's Other Planet: Israeli Youth Imagine the Holocaust", *Jewish Social Studies 3:2* (1997), 42–76.

Ben-Gurion, Emanuel, "House of Dolls", *Davar*, 12 April 1953. [Hebrew].

Bertini, Aharon K., *Gilyonot,* March–April (1953). [Hebrew].

Breuer, Josef and Freud, Sigmund, *Studies on Hysteria*, ed. and trans. James Strachey (Hogarth Press, 1955).

Calinescu, Matel, *Faces of Modernity, Avant-Garde, Decadence, Kitsch* (Duke University Press, 1987).

Caruth, Cathy, ed., *Trauma: Explorations in Memory* (Johns Hopkins UP, 1995).

Cohen, Uri S., "Ka-Tzetnik, Primo Levi, and the Muslims", in Annette F. Timm, ed., *Holocaust History and the Reading of Ka-Tzetnik* (Bloomsbury, 2018), 153–166.

Dinur, Yehiel, "I Accuse", *Bamahaneh*, May 1961. [Hebrew].

Dinur, Yehiel, https://www.youtube.com/watch?v=m3-tXyYhd5U

Dror, Zvika, "Nightmare Holds Him in Its Grip", *Massa Davar*, 20 April 1990. [Hebrew].

Dudai, Rina, *Modes of Coping with Trauma in Holocaust Literature* (Doctoral thesis. Hebrew University, 2000). [Hebrew].

Dudai, Rina, "Kitsch and Trauma: A Reading of Ka-tzetnik's *House of Dolls*", *Mikan 6* (2006) 125–146. [Hebrew].

Dudai, Rina, "Pain and Pleasure in Poetic Representations of the Holocaust", in Amos Goldberg and Haim Hazan, eds., *Marking Evil, Holocaust Memory in the Global Age* (Berghahn, 2015), 233–265.

Evans, Dylan, *An Introductory Dictionary of Lacanian Psychoanalysis* (Routledge, 1986).

Felman, Shoshana, *The Juridical Unconscious* (Harvard UP, 2002).

Freud, Sigmund, "Beyond the Pleasure Principle", in James Strachey, ed. and trans., *The Standard Edition of the Complete Psychological Works, Vol. 18* (Hogarth Press, 2001), 7–66.

Freud, Sigmund, "Mourning and Melancholia", in James Strachey, ed. and trans., *The Standard Edition of the Complete Psychological Works, Vol. 14: On the History of the*

Psycho-Analytic Movement, Papers on Metapsychology and Other Works (Hogarth Press, 2001), 243–258.
Friedländer, Saul, *Reflections of Nazism*, trans. Thomas Weyer (Harper & Row, [1982] 1984).
Friedländer, Saul, ed., *Probing the Limits of Representation: Nazism and the Final Solution* (Harvard University Press, 1992).
Glasner-Heled, Galia, "Who Does Ka-Tzetnik Represent?" *Dapim 20* (2005), 190. [Hebrew].
Goldberg, Amos, *Trauma in First-Person: Diary Writing during the Holocaust* (Indiana University Press, 2017).
Goldberg, Amos and Hazan, Haim, eds., *Marking Evil, Holocaust Memory in the Global Age* (Berghahn, 2015).
Grinwald, Itamar, Collins, Adela Yarbro, Mitchell, Margaret Mary, and Betz, Hans-Dieter, "Paul and Ritual Theory: The Case of 'The Lord's Supper' in 1 Corinthians 10 and 11", in Collins Adela Yarbro and Mitchel Margaret Mary, eds., *Antiquity and Humanity: Essays on Ancient Religion and Philosophy* (Mohr Siebeck, 2001), 159–187.
Halamish, M., "The Clock Overhead", *Al Hamishmar*, 20 January 1961. [Hebrew].
Ka-Tzetnik, *House of Dolls*, trans. Moshe M. Kohn (Simon and Schuster, [1953] 1955).
Ka-Tzetnik, *Ha'Tzofen* (Kibbutz Meuchad, [1987] 1991), 85 [Hebrew].
Keshet, Yeshurun, "Dolls House by Ka-Tzetnik", *Davar*, 27 February 1953. [Hebrew].
Kristeva, Julia, *Powers of Horror: An Essay on Abjection*, trans. Roudiez Leon (Columbia University Press, 1982).
Kulka, Tomas, ed., *Kitsch and Art* (Penn State University Press, 1996).
Kundera, Milan, "*The Unbearable Lightness of Being*", trans. Michael Henry Heim [Harper Perennial, [1984] 2009].
Lacan, Jacques and Mehlman, Jeffrey, "Seminar on the 'Purloined Letter'", *Yale French Studies 48* (1972), 39–72.
Lambert, Wilfred G. and Parker, Simon B., *Enûma Eliš. The Babylonian Epic of Creation* (Oxford, 1966). Tab. 1: 134–145.
Lander, P., "The Girl from the House of Dolls", *Haaretz*, 16 October 1953. [Hebrew].
Laub, Dori, "Bearing Witness or the Vicissitudes of Listening", in Shoshana Felman and Dori Laub, eds., *Testimony: Crises of Witnessing in Literature, Psychoanalysis, and History* (Routledge, 1992), 57–74.
Longinus, *Longinus on the Sublime*, trans. W. Rhys Robert (Cambridge University Press, 1907), Chapter 12, 77.
Lyotard, Jean-Francois, *The Differend: Phrases in Dispute*, trans. Abbeele George Van Den (University of Minnesota Press, [1983] 1988), 22–23.
Miller, Jacques-Alain, *Le partenaire-symptôme: l'orientation lacanienne, 1997–1998* (Martinière, 2003).
Milner, Iris, "The Evil Spirits of the Shoah: Ka-Tzetnik's Literary Testimony to Death and Survival in the Concentrationary Universe", in Annette F. Timm, ed., *Holocaust History and the Reading of Ka-Tzetnik* (Bloomsbury, 2018), 67–78.
Miron, Dan, "Between Book and Ashes", *Alpayim 10* (1995), 196–224. [Hebrew].
Nahor, Asher, "The House of Dolls", *Herut*, 6 March 1953. [Hebrew].
Nozick, Robert, "On Kitsch", in Kulka Tomas, ed., *Kitsch and Art* (Penn State University Press, 1996), 99.
Pelli, Moshe, "The Art of Ka-Tzetnik's Type of Holocaust Literature", *Mahut 2* (1990), 148–159. [Hebrew].

Reuveni, Yotam, "Salamandra", *Ot*, 12 January 1972. [Hebrew].
Santner, Eric L., "History beyond the Pleasure Principle: Some Thoughts on the Representation of Trauma", in Saul Friedländer, ed., *Probing the Limits of Representation: Nazism and the Final Solution* (Harvard University Press, 1992), 143–154.
Segev, Tom, *The Seventh Million: The Israelis and the Holocaust*, trans. Haim Watzman (Picador, 2000), 4.
Sheintokh, Yehiel, *Innocent Speaker: Conversations with Yehiel Dinur* (Bet Lohamey Hageta'ot, Dov Sadan Institute, 2003).
Sheintokh, Yechiel, *Salamandra: Myth and History* (Carmel, 2009), 31–34. [Hebrew].
Shofman, Gershon, "Salamandra", *Davar*, 20 December 1946. [Hebrew].
Talpaz, Gideon, "Trilogy of Death", *Davar*, 11 August 1977. [Hebrew].
Timm, Annette F., ed., *Holocaust History and the Reading of Ka-Tzetnik* (Bloomsbury, 2018), 67–78.
Vanier, Alain, *Lacan* (Other Press, 2000).
White, Hayden, "The Value of Narrativity in the Representation of Reality", *Critical Inquiry 7:1* (1980), 5–27.
White, Hayden, "Historiography as Narration", in Joseph Smith and Morris Humphrey, eds., *Telling Facts: History and Narration in Psychoanalysis* (Johns Hopkins University Press, 1992), 284–299.
Yaffe, Mordechai, "On 'House of Dolls'", *Al Hamishmar*, 6 June 1958. [Hebrew].

Chapter 5

On Rational Traumatic Memory in Primo Levi's *If This Is a Man* and Other Works

Primo Levi – A Biographical Sketch

Primo Levi was born on July 31, 1919 in Turin, Italy, in an established, assimilated Jewish family. During his adolescence the Fascist Party ruled Italy; he began his studies at the Institute of Chemistry at Turin University in 1937 and graduated in 1941 even though by that point racial legislation had been introduced. When, in July 1943, Mussolini temporarily lost power and the Germans invaded, Levi joined the underground movement *Giustizia e Liberta.* He and other comrades were betrayed and captured on December 13, 1943. Levi, who confessed his Jewish identity, was sent to Fossoli near Modena, and from there he was put on a train to Auschwitz. On February 26, 1944, at his arrival in the extermination camp, prisoner number 174517 was tattooed onto his arm. Soviet soldiers liberated the camp on January 27, 1945, and on October 19 that year, after a long, arduous journey which he described in *The Truce* (1965), he returned to Turin. He started a family and began working at the SIVA paints factory, to eventually become its director. At the same time, while pursuing his career as a chemist, he wrote and published his literary works, which are also autobiographical documents.

When he retired from his work at SIVA, in 1975, Levi planned to dedicate himself his writing. His literary work had gained an international reputation over the years, but he suffered from writer's block and depression. In an interview not long before his death, he complained that he had written at least three books while working as a chemist, yet later on, when he made time for writing, he ended up writing less and with less intensity.[1] Levi underwent relatively successful surgery to remove a cancerous growth but was left to cope with persistent complications. He committed suicide on April 11, 1987.[2]

His Father's Heritage

In his writings, Levi mentioned how strongly he had been influenced by his father, Cesare Levi, especially in two regards: the repressed terror underlying Jewish existence and a deep attachment and commitment to Enlightenment values. His father, an engineer who had worked in France and Hungary for long stints, had

DOI: 10.4324/9781003403753-8

experienced antisemitism and had witnessed Bela Kun's 1919 coup d'état in Budapest. He talked very little with his son about these things.[3] It was mainly through literature and his love of science that Levi, the father, passed his Enlightenment values to his son. In his essay "The Invisible World,"[4] Levi recounts how, when he was 15 years old, his father gave him an old English book, published in 1846, entitled *Thoughts on Animalcules; or, A Glimpse of the Invisible World Revealed by the Microscope*.[5] Levi did not know English, so he bought a dictionary and got immersed, much more enthusiastically than when reading the mandatory literature on the high school curriculum. When he asked for a microscope, his father bought him one as well as an etymological dictionary to satisfy his curiosity about the history of words.[6]

During his high school years, it was linguistics rather than literature that interested Levi. But he acquired a profound familiarity with the literary classics, like Aristotle, Dante, and Leopardi.[7] By age 14, he had made up his mind to become a chemist. Science, for him, was a poetic discipline: chemistry, as he saw it, was no less poetic than the *Divine Comedy*, and university studies appeared to him a sanctuary of reason and logic amid the madness of fascism. Clarity and precision, later, would be a hallmark of his writing. And so, Levi developed a strong intellectual bent in which reason functioned as the main tool for looking at the world.

Enlightenment as Ideal

Though he did not identify himself as an intellectual, the worldview reflected in *If This Is a Man*, as well as in later work, meets the criteria he himself proposed in his book *The Drowned and the Saved* (1986). He proposed that an intellectual can be defined as someone educated beyond his profession, who continuously expands his knowledge and remains open to new fields without indifference or frustration, even if he cannot master them all.[8]

In Levi's educational and cultural environment, humanistic and scientific values in the spirit of the European Enlightenment coexisted harmoniously. Kant had defined Enlightenment as leaving behind a state of immaturity: the truly critical and therefore enlightened mind only emerges when human thought is autonomous and free from the shackles of emotion, the pressures of institutions (like religion), from prejudice and superstition. "Dare to know" is Kant's challenge to the mature individual: "Have the courage to use your intelligence!"[9] For Kant, therefore, liberation is from the irrational forces we encounter, originating from both inside ourselves and outside. Levi, too, mentioned that the power of reason gave him his most sublime sense of freedom in the midst of the most irrational of experiences.

Auschwitz, for Levi, was a trial of human reason. Admitting that reason did not help when it came to physical survival – Enlightenment man found himself at a disadvantage in the face of hard labor –paradoxically, it was at the site of greatest violence that he most keenly felt a need for culture. It was culture that helped him maintain a connection with the past, rescue it from oblivion, protecting, thereby, his very identity.[10] In addition to the store of knowledge with which he entered the camp, he was also equipped with certain habits of thought and analysis, questions of the kind asked in science, like if he acts in a certain way, how will the substance he holds in his hands react, or his human interlocutor?[11] Auschwitz, therefore, presented him with a demanding experience, intellectually speaking.

Levi and Language

Enlightenment reason, science, and social perceptions share a faith in the role of language. In Levi's case this finds expression on three levels: language has the power to bring order to chaos; it is responsible for communication, and it represents culture. In his article "On Obscure Writing,"[12] Levi formulated an unambiguous demand for clear and transparent language. This need for precision and accuracy derived from his education in chemistry. For him scientific accuracy was the most reliable mode of describing, understanding, and exposing reality, even when he wrote literary texts.

He rejected the common equation between authentic writing and writing "from the heart." It was an approach, he believed, that stems from the misperception that heart and reason are two different entities, with the heart featuring as more noble. Levi argues that the language of the heart is capricious, tainted, and unreliable. In fact, it is not a language at all, qualifying rather as idiom or jargon, an idiosyncrasy.

Of course, Levi acknowledges that some people write to relieve tension, alleviate pain, or express joy, when the author "cries in the desert," as he puts it.[13] But the desert, for him, is essentially the domain of the unintelligible, the site of what comes before language, and sobbing is the outlet for the individual's tears, not an expression in language. It was Levi's life mission to convey what he experienced in Auschwitz in clear and distinct words, thereby setting it free from barbarism. In doing so, he brought to bear the cultural roots of the Enlightenment, which required him to bring order to chaos, using rational language.

Language as a Means of Communication

For Levi the communicative aspect of language is meaningful in terms of survival, in relation to both the concrete conditions of the extermination camp as well as in terms of writing about the experience.

In an interview, Levi mentioned three basic traumas he associated with the camp, all of them involving language: the absence of solidarity, the absence of communication, and violence.[14] Levi had the good fortune of knowing some German, acquired when he studied chemistry. This enabled him to form a somewhat better idea of what the place was like. A great many languages were spoken in the camp, and this impeded communication, amplifying the lack of solidarity. The ability to communicate was an existential sine qua non in these circumstances.[15] Levi believed that one of the main causes of prisoners' death was unfamiliarity with the language.

Levi does not only discuss language in so far as it is a possibly life-saving tool of communication but also as what allows him to write about the events in the camp. The reader, for Levi, has a contract with the writer: when the reader does not understand the text, this amounts to an offense; it is deceit. The overriding importance of communication – passing on information or emotions from one place to another, from one person to another, from one moment to another – makes clarity of the essence. But if the reader did not understand the writer, or would feel unjustly humiliated, the writer would be guilty of a breach of contract.[16]

Alongside the demand for clarity, Levi also insists on exchange and communication, even with the enemy, the perpetrator. A German publisher acquired the translation rights of *If This Is a Man*, and this translation was the occasion of writing the eighth chapter of *The Drowned and the Saved*: letters written by German readers to Levi and his responses to them. Many of the prisoners in the extermination camps developed a hatred of the German language, which they came to see as the language of death, but Levi made a distinction. The cultural tolerance he had imbibed from the history of the Italian language translated, for him, into a cultural position. He realized that the German of the Lager – skeletal, howled, studded with obscenities and imprecations – was vaguely related to the precise language of his chemistry books or to the melodious, refined German of Heine's poetry. His observation on the language in the camp was that where violence is inflicted on man, it is also inflicted on language.[17]

Language as Cultural Tool

Language helped Levi connect to his cultural roots – Jewish, Italian, and Western in general. It is his attachment to language that enabled him to stay sane. He began his book *The Periodic Table* (1975)[18] with a chapter entitled "Argon," which consists of a small history of the dialect of the Jews of Italy's Piedmont region. Writing this chapter, in the 1970s, Levi had a choice of three languages: Italian, the Piedmontese dialect, and the Jewish-Piedmontese dialect. Of these three, the last is the most esoteric, but Levi chose it.

In Chapter 6 of *The Drowned and the Saved*, which discusses the intellectual in Auschwitz, Levi refers to his chapter, "The Canto of Ulysses," in *If This Is a Man*, where he described his attempt at recollecting Dante's "Inferno," to translate it to a French co-prisoner who did not know Italian. This act of recollection and the subsequent translation of the text come to preserve historical-cultural continuity. In doing so Levi joins the cultural chain leading through Odysseus and Dante.[19]

For Levi, science, like literature, is in the domain of the sublime. What they have in common is reason, which for Levi equals what divine grace means for Christians. For a non-believer like himself, reason is the one power that can help make sense of the world, thereby advancing progress towards a better, more whole world. Reason supports an optimistic vision of human redemption. The pleasure of the sublime, according to Levi, is Kantian in nature and derives from the triumph of reason over the senses and fantasy.[20] Levi's most sublime experience during his time in Auschwitz, the most barbarous place in the world, occurred when he had a near mystical experience of reason as what sets humans apart from all other life on earth. He achieved this moment when, as mentioned above, he rehearsed and translated "The Canto of Ulysses," insisting on maintaining cultural continuity.[21]

Language as a Tool for Poetic Writing

The Holocaust became the formative event of Levi's life. Unlike his friend, Jean Améry, for whom, according to Levi, Auschwitz did not serve as a source of knowledge,[22] Levi himself thought of Auschwitz as a place, however cruel, where something new was to be learned. The Lager was for him a university.[23] The experience was what drove his entire oeuvre. Like the ancient mariner in Coleridge's "Ballad of the Ancient Mariner," it burned inside him until he died: "And till my ghastly tale is told/ This heart within me burns."[24]

If This Is a Man (*Se Questo e un Uomo*, 1947, 1958) was Levi's first book, and he wrote it immediately upon returning to Turin. It was a personal account, not a novel. He set out to write it without a plan, with a sense of obligation towards his dead friends and to render his recent, searing memories. The first draft consisted of fourteen pages describing the final days of Auschwitz. They eventually became the last chapter of the book. It took Levi a few months to complete the manuscript and look for a publisher. While some selected chapters were published in a Communist newspaper in the course of 1946, the manuscript was rejected by all major publishing houses. In the autumn of 1947, 2500 copies were published (privately) and mainly distributed among relatives and friends. Levi was so disappointed that he hardly wrote anything other than a few short stories until 1961. There was a reprint of *If This Is a Man*, including some new background material in June 1958, consisting of a cautious 2000 copies. This time, too, the book seemed to vanish into a black hole.

In December 1961, Levi was asked to write about his return home. The book, *The Truce* (*La Tregua*),[25] was published in April 1963 and was an immediate success. This epic of Levi's return from the forests and swamps of Belarus to Turin, via Ukraine, Romania, Hungary, Austria, and Germany, conveyed his sense of liberation at the end of his year in Auschwitz. This is what Levi said about writing *The Truce*: "When I wrote *The Truce* I chose the clearest possible language, in the hope the information would come through without distortion to the reader."[26]

As said, in contrast with *If This Is a Man*, *The Truce* was an almost overnight success. Critics praised the author's clear language and his historical and moral perceptions, as well as the book's picaresque structure, its humor, pace, and moments of hope. The enthusiastic reception also meant a turning point in Levi's life: he was no longer read merely as a "Holocaust writer."[27] In 1965, *If This Is a Man* and *The Truce* came out in one volume, and the book became part of the Italian curriculum in 1973. The two works were very popular among young readers.[28]

The initial difference in readers' responses to these two texts has two possible reasons. The first involves the general public's readiness to deal with the subject matter. *If This Is a Man* describes the heart of darkness. Levi, who had been there, recounted his story, but just like in a frequent nightmare he had, the readers were not ready yet to hear it. With *The Truce*, which describes Levi's personal odyssey, this was different. The audience wanted, and got, a happy ending, with the hero returning home. The second reason for these different reception trajectories concerns the lapse of time: Written in 1945 and first published in 1947, a mere two years after the war, *If This Is a Man* met with a readership still in the grip of shock and denial. By the time *The Truce* was published in 1963, eighteen years had passed, long enough for the Holocaust to have undergone some processing, and the fact that this work described the road to rehabilitation rather than the horror itself helped along.

During the 1970s Primo Levi became a public figure. He left his career in chemistry to dedicate himself to *The Periodic Table* (*Il Sistema Periodica*, 1975). On its publication in 1975, Levi found himself one of Italy's most prominent contemporary writers. The book is dominated by the intellectual effort of penetrating how chemical change occurs due to the combination of substances. Chemistry functions as a metaphor of life.[29] *The Periodic Table* displays Levi's love of condensation, in both the chemical and the literary sense, and his wish to penetrate the nature of processes of assimilation, liberation, and change. These he saw as crucial points of connection between scientific reality and the artistic imagination, as well as, eventually, a major tool for interpreting the world.

The book takes two main formats: the literary genre of autobiography and the scientific structure of Mendeleev's periodic table. Levi presents his family history and the formative events in his own life over the course of twenty-one chapters – following the paradigm of the periodic table. The order is biographical-chronological, starting from Levi's ancestors, through life in the Italy of Mussolini, the years of Levi's rehabilitation, and the 1960s, and his extraordinary correspondence with the German Dr. Müller, with whom he worked in the camp's lab. The book concludes with a meditation on the chemical process of writing.

In 1975, a collection of his poems, *Collected Poems* (*L'osteria di Brema*), was published, followed, in 1984, by another one: *Collected Poems* (*Ad ora incerta*),[30] a title referring to Coleridge's earlier mentioned poem. Levi called himself an occasional poet (he wrote about one poem a year). In addition, he published further books of prose: *The Wrench* (*La Chiave a Stella*, 1978);[31] *If Not Now, When?* (*Se non ora, Quando*, 1982);[32] *Other People's Trades* (*L'altrui Mestiere*, 1985);[33] *The Drowned and the Saved* (*I sommersi e I salvati*, 1986);[34] and *The Mirror Maker* (*Racconti e Saggi*, 1986).[35]

The Drowned and the Saved consists of eight articles dedicated to a critical examination of historical, psychological, and artistic representations of traumatic experiences. Here he considers the inevitability of oblivion; the "grey zone" of collaboration between victims and perpetrators; the persistent shame of the liberated prisoner; the anguish of not having died: and the way in which the victim, unwillingly and blamelessly, turns into a collaborator in the scene of horror. The Italian for "drowned" – *sommersi* – is a reference to Dante's "Inferno,"[36] where it denotes the cursed masses who are dead both physically and mentally. Many have wondered whether there is some connection between this book, which first appeared a year before his death, and Levi's suicide, and whether it should be read as his testament.[37]

The Mystery of the Centaur: The Split World

Having dedicated his life to two very disparate disciplines – science and literature – Levi was always interested in forging a link between them. Drawing on Galileo, who had a unified and undivided culture, he claimed that there should be one single culture.[38] This seems to express a wish to speak in one language, blending between the discourses of science and literature. Yet, nevertheless he experienced himself as "split in two":

> I am amphibian, a *centaur* (I've even written stories about centaurs) [...] I am split in two. One half of me is of the factory, is the technician and the chemist, but there is another, quite separate half that lives in the world of writing [...] They are two parts of me that exist [...] distinctly [...].[39]

Here I will adopt the image of the centaur[40] as a kind of prism through which I look at the interrelationship in Levi's work between the instinctual and emotional world of writing, on the one hand, and the rational-scientific, on the other. Did Levi achieve this fusion? Below I will reflect on the tension between feeling, not admitted under the sway of reason, and the way it, nevertheless, breaks through.

Let us briefly dwell on the figure of the centaur. The centaur, part man and part horse, is one of the chimeras,[41] hybrid creatures composed of different animal parts, all figures from Greek mythology. The chimeras have an important mythopoetic function, as they undo the fixed hierarchy between human, animal, and divine by creating a new hybrid creature. Centaurs – the best known among them are Nessus and Pollux – usually described in Greek mythology as wild and cruel, symbolizing lawlessness and passion. The struggle between the Centaurs and Lapiths, in which the latter's reason gained the upper hand over the former's barbarousness, accumulated important metaphorical meaning, and became a commonplace of Greek art.

In his short story, "Quaestio de Centauris,"[42] which first appeared in the periodical *Il Mundo* on April 4, 1961, Levi is inspired by this myth. This fantasy story is about the fusion between man and horse in paradise and how the expulsion from paradise leads the centaur into the world. The exile from paradise, in this story, reveals the impossibility, in our actual world, of hybridity.[43] Exiled from paradise, the creature in which the human and the animal had harmoniously dwelled together splits into drives and reason, forming an unstable compound, always on the verge of disintegration.[44]

The story opens with a centaur being kept in a stall by the narrator's father, who didn't know where else to keep him. He had received the centaur from a friend – a sea captain – who claimed to have bought him in Salonika. The narrator, however, later learns directly from his father's friend that he was actually born in Colophon.[45]

Colophon was a Greek city in Asia Minor, not far from present-day Izmir in Turkey, but the name also refers to an inscription at the end of a book or manuscript carrying the title or subject of the work, its author, the name of the printer or publisher, and date and place of publication. Often the colophon received special attention in terms of style and graphics.[46] That Levi mentioned Colophon, therefore, suggests that the story, over and beyond being about the reciprocities between man and animal, also refers to the relations between the universe of the book and reality outside it, between the world of myth and the imagination, and the actual world. This hybridity, in Levi's story, is played out between two narrative voices: One is that of an omniscient narrator, who didactically offers semantic information about centaurs, as though this was an encyclopedic project. The other narrator presents a personal account of a recollected and formative coming-of-age experience. These transitions in style produce a hesitant effect – one of the characteristics of the genre of fantasy, according to Todorov[47] – an oscillation between fantasy or fiction and actual reality. The narrators in Levi's story blend together, with the didactic tone dominating initially and later the more personal. The story ends by opening out into a tale recounted by a group of fishermen who briefly glimpsed a man riding a dolphin, or perhaps a transformed centaur, who then disappeared.

The omniscient narrator offers a story about the centaur unlike the versions common in Greek mythology. His account refers to the Biblical myth of the deluge and the Ark of Noah, and he forges a tale about a *second creation*. When the waters receded, a thick layer of warm mud was left behind, covering the earth. From this mud a rich variety of creatures sprang.

The second creation, therefore, occurred at the end of the dystopian era, an inaugurating event after the catastrophe, rejecting destruction and death, under the sign of love among the species. Since it generated these hybrid fusions, the narrator calls this "true creation." The warm mud is the cradle for the entire universe. The narrator zooms in on the appearance of the centaurs, powerful, noble creatures in whom the best of human and horse, respectively, come together. They are wise and brave, generous and intelligent, sensitive and remarkably perceptive.

The plot about Trachi, the centaur, starts only halfway into the story. This is when the omniscient narrator is replaced by the experiencing narrator, who recounts his episodic recollections, a personal story about himself and Trachi, with whom he grew up secretly, out of the sight of envious strangers. Trachi's most conspicuous attribute, in this description, is his extraordinary ability to register the smallest nuances in nature. He can feel a storm approaching hours before it arrives, for instance, and senses any sexual activity in his surroundings.

The tragic ending of this story, cryptically referring to the lost fantasy, is apparent before the narrative properly sets off. One summer, the narrator falls in love with Teresa De Simone, his neighbor, who left home and returns as a young adult. The narrator, Teresa De Simone, and Trachi spend a wonderful, unforgettable evening together. The next morning the centaur tells the narrator that he has fallen in love with Teresa. He is aware of the impossibility of this love, but, still, he yearns for her alone. His soul has turned into a battlefield in which his violent, primitive ancestors, Nessus and Pollux, have taken over while his other, human part is overcome by omnipotent heroic dreams of a second creation. One night, the narrator and Teresa sleep together, and on returning home, they find that Trachi is gone. While they were making love, he galloped away into the distance. On his wild rampage he attacked mares and wreaked destruction. The story concludes like a legend, and Trachi is never seen again.

Following the long introduction, told by the omniscient narrator, and just prior to the start of the plot, narrated in the first-person singular, Levi pauses for a non-diegetic reflection – i.e., a reflection situated outside the story's main narrative – on the act of writing itself. He confesses that writing about this episode is a painful activity and lets us know that in the very act of writing, or of telling the story, he departs from a passionate experience whose realization turns out to have been impossible: "It pains me to write this story. It is a story from my youth, and I feel as if in writing it I were expelling it from myself, and later I will feel deprived of something strong and pure."[48]

This interpellation is a formative, though painful, moment in Levi's writing. The pain is two-fold: In terms of the narrative as such, the symbiotic moment, situated in the remote past of the second creation, when reason and feeling became fused within the centaur – this moment is forever gone. In terms of the very act of writing, which processes the experience, Levi casts out intense emotion and precious experience, thus depriving himself of his very essence. Here, almost unnoticeably, Levy enfolds an important comment on what it means to be writing on trauma.

When, at the end of the story, the centaur, overcome with love, leaves his hiding place, he faces a cruel reality: the fantasy of fusion and a return to the era of second creation are no longer possible. Paradise has collapsed, and he is left vulnerable and frustrated. Now a violence that annihilates everything that crosses his path erupts from him. At the end of the story, the boundaries between author, narrator, and protagonist, Trachi, the hybrid creature, also come undone. Only the fishermen remain to bear witness to a man riding the back of a dolphin, vanishing among the waves.

I would like to argue that Levi, the centaur, made a huge effort throughout his life as a writer to rein in the horse-like element he carried within him by imposing the power of human reason. For him, accurate scientific writing, devoid of feeling, came to set off the outburst of instinct: this would bridle the destructiveness triumphant at the end of the centaur's story.

Rational Restraint

Levi's literary writing, as he himself put it, was like a weekly business or laboratory report.[49] He was indeed most deeply versed in scientific method and discourse.[50]

The first thing he wrote, as soon as he was liberated from Auschwitz in January 1945, was a report, invited by the USSR military command, on the hygienic-medical organization of the camp, which he co-authored with the camp surgeon, Leonardo de Benedetti.[51] The resulting text is a great effort at objectivity. Testimony is detached and restrained; the style is cautious and measured: all in order to describe with utmost precision, and without getting emotional, the inhuman practices to which the author had fallen victim. The report detailed the illnesses in the camp and described the clinics treating them, the shortage of medicine, and the lack of hygienic conditions. It concludes with a description of the selection of Muselmanns and the operation of the gas chambers, offering a detailed and painstakingly objective survey of the way the victims were murdered.

In *If This Is a Man*, first published in 1947, Levi again portrayed Auschwitz from the researcher's perspective. Below I call the manner in which Levi brings order to chaos *rational restraint*.

Rational Restraint in *If This Is a Man*

> I adopted a dense and accurate style, allowing for no excess. The habit of carefully considering every word and avoiding imprecise expression, originates in the demands of, and my inclination toward, the science laboratory. I wanted to bring back things from memory, describe them with utmost precision and lacking any excess burden or cliché. The horror needed no highlighting – it inheres in everything I recount.[52]

Speaking here in Karl William's documentary film "Primo Levi," Levi mentioned two main elements of his writing: it shuns anything superfluous, and it does not leave out anything. In another interview, shortly before his death, Levi said this to Roberto Di Caro: "The decisive element for narrative procedure is a careful balance between the essential and the superfluous [...]."[53]

I will discuss this controlled and restrained balance in the context of the rationalist worldview I have presented above. I believe that it forms the intellectual as well as the psychological foundation of Levi's stylistic predilections. I consider Levi's literary style in *If This Is a Man*, which is one of the most exceptional documents about Auschwitz. Levi limited himself strictly to what he had seen, to what he knew, and to how he understood these things in his context. Describing the people, conditions, objects, and events, Levi rendered the discursive space of the impossible, between life and death.

Dissociation Yielding Differentiation

Seeking to achieve maximum accuracy, Levi chose a restrained, perspicacious, and sharp mode of representation. This approach he develops mainly by means of a mechanism that causes dissociation or splitting while contemplating the traumatic experience. This mechanism allows him to examine the traumatic event from various perspectives, thus to creating a distinct and complex reconstruction of reality; the observer is kept at a remove from the intensity of experience. Here I will discuss three types of splitting: splitting achieved through changes of location within the camp, splitting originating in a change of function, and splitting between scientific and poetic modes.

Splitting was achieved through changes of location within the extermination camp: When during a day of exhausting labor, Levi injured his foot, he decided to go to the *Ka-Be*, short for *Krankenbau*, i.e., the camp infirmary. This results in a change of location that affords Levi a different perspective on where he is. It is as if waking from a dream he finds himself in a different state of consciousness. It was like a returning from nothingness.[54] He hears the orchestra starting to play in the distance, knowing that those of his friends who are (still) healthy are setting off to work. From where he is in the *Ka-Be*, he imagines them like robots marching to the sound of satanic music.[55]

Levi was all too familiar with this daily road of tribulations to and from harsh forced labor, but it required a change of location within this infernal setting to gain a different, more conscious angle. Through long days of inaction, inmates of the Ka-Be began to experience a change within. He started to reflect on what they had turned them into, how much they had taken away from them, and what this life had become.[56]

The movement from the regular prisoners' barracks to the infirmary produced, in Levi, a split way of looking at the camp, as if from an external vantage point that allowed reflection. Away from physical abuse and torture, his consciousness was as it were stirred, showing him reality in its stark outlines.

When he is moved to a new workplace, Dr. Pannwitz's chemical laboratory, the effect is similar. The three people who are selected to work there on grounds of their professional expertise are thus sentenced to live. The laboratory staff, though indifferent, are, at least, not hostile. The place is properly heated, and conditions are more relaxed. Now, they no longer suffer hunger either. And much like in the case of Levi's temporary move to the Ka-Be, here too, once physical discomfort is reduced and the spatial reference point changes, Levi sees things differently, more reflectively. This time his observations include recollections from times before the camp. Not only does the change of work open a possibility to contemplate the camp's cruel reality, it broadens consciousness, making it possible for Levi to access his inner world, his dreams and thoughts, beyond the material here and now of a horrifying reality.

Splitting Originating in a Change of Function

In the chapter "Initiation," Levi mentions how much the Germans were attached to hygiene, and that most public announcements in the camp involved orders to stay clean. This emphasis on cleanliness cohered with received ideas about German attitudes to hygiene, and in Levi it triggered a contrary impulse. He confesses that it gave him a sense of minimal human freedom, or agency, when he saved some time by *not washing*. He wonders about the point of washing. Will it make him feel better? Will he appear more pleasant to anyone? Will it replenish his strength?

What he cares about is only how to preserve as much energy for the next cruel task awaiting him.

His friend Steinlauf sees things very differently. He explains that since the camp's objective is to turn them into beasts, they must do everything they can to avoid turning into exactly that. Steinlauf agrees with Levi that even though they are slaves shorn of all rights, whom the Nazis are free to humiliate, insult, and eventually kill, they maintain some ability not to consent. This is why they must wash their faces and polish their shoes: not because that's what they have been ordered to do, but to stay alive, not to begin to die.[57]

Steinlauf takes an existentialist view of their desperate reality – reminiscent of what Albert Camus described in *The Myth of Sisyphus*.[58] Sisyphus, according to Camus, does not alter anything in the world. Reality stays untransformed: A tall mountain; a rock that must be pushed up the slope; Sisyphus, who is doomed to perform this labor. Sisyphus's heroism inheres in his redefining his relationship to the world. He refuses to be the rock's object: instead, the rock becomes his. Taking responsibility and embracing his fate, he adds vitality and meaning to his life.

Levi, however, is not convinced. The chapter concludes with him formulating his doubts. This split perspective produces different ways of looking at the function of washing.

Splitting into Scientific and Poetic Modes

Levi, the scientist, looked at Auschwitz as an experiment at humanity under extreme pressure. This allowed him to investigate, as through a process of distillation, the essential components of a human being. This is among other things, why the book is titled *If This Is a Man*:

> We would also like to consider that the Lager was pre-eminently a gigantic biological and social experiment. Thousands of individuals, differing in age, condition, origin, language, culture and customs, are enclosed within barbed wire: there they live a regular, controlled life which is identical for all and inadequate to all needs, and which is more rigorous than any experimenter could have set up to establish what is essential and what adventitious to the conduct of the human animal in the struggle for life.[59]

Levi's laboratory paradigm can be seen to replace Ka-tzetnik's paradigm of the other planet, "Kokhav Haefer" (Star of Ashes). Presenting a two-fold representation, literal and metaphoric simultaneously, the paradigm is complex. In some literal and concrete sense, it is indeed possible to gain sociological, psychological, and biological data from this multi-dimensional experiment. At the same time however, we can understand it metaphorically: here humans are in the role of experimental mice, presenting us with human behaviors under stressful conditions. Unlike Ka-Tzetnik's central metaphor, which takes both him and his readers into apocalyptic dimensions, this one maintains a connection with reality.

If This Is a Man reflects Levi's scientific literacy. Science differs from other ways of knowing in the characteristics and standards that define and delimit its practical domain, its methods of realization, and its response to reality. The scientific method relies on modes of action and thinking that include methodical observation, quantification and organization of data, drawing empirical conclusions for the sake of theory construction, questioning existing theories, and constant re-examination against empirical reality by means of either rational or physical tests.[60]

Explanations of the world can be grounded in myth, religion, a variety of beliefs, prejudices, or schemata. All of these are conceptually as well as practically unlike science insofar as they do not base their knowledge on methodical testing and confirmation against empirical reality, and do not engage in fundamentally skeptical and non-authoritarian negotiations with that reality. His scientific experience deeply affected Levi's literary writing. It is owing to his background in chemistry that this writing is marked by accuracy and restraint, chemistry being the art of isolation, weighing, and analysis, all necessary when a person wishes to describe a phenomenon, Levi thought. Unsurprisingly, therefore, the observations of Levi, the scientist, characteristically sought for connections and attempted to create order in even the most extreme, chaotic experiences. It was the scientific method and deduction that offered him a stability shielding him from the shock of surprise.

Levi considered it his task as both a chemist and a writer, to forge a path leading out of the dark and into light, from chaos to order. This is how he put it in *The Periodic Table* when he spoke about struggling in darkness, feeling lost, until a faint light appears, growing stronger, and order finally emerges from chaos.[61] The classic Enlightenment metaphor, the escape from darkness to light, is easily identified in Levy's writing: it expresses an optimistic approach, putting faith in both science and poetry.

One notable activity in scientific work is classification, that is, the methodical arrangement of phenomena in hierarchical-categorical terms. This methodical classification can clearly be seen at work in Levi's chapter on "The Drowned and the Saved" in *If This is a Man*.[62] Here Levi examines the characters he observes in the camp and presents them deductively – starting from generalization and moving forward into details and exemplification. Levi distinguishes between two particularly well-differentiated categories among men – the drowned and the saved.[63] Those who are sentenced to death all share the same trait, namely that they are Muselmanns even before properly turning into them. Their progress is staked out from the start, and their end is foretold.[64]

The second type, the saved, Levi categorizes into four sub-types, and he describes them at length: Schepschel; Alfred L., the engineer, with his rigid style and discipline, who anticipated things and made himself into a civil servant long before actually becoming one; Elias Lindzin, the dwarf, who had a personality radiating animal strength and was unstoppable; and Henry, a man of culture, a survivor who excelled at deceit and theft.[65]

Levi's scientific tendencies are also evident in his accurate, minimalist formulations. The book features a great deal of quantitative reporting, couched in a factual mode of narration. This feature also is behind the powerful restraint in his communication of the extremely charged material. This is how he describes the fateful moment of selection, when his life briefly hangs in the balance: “In three or four minutes a hut of two hundred men is ‘done’, as is the whole camp of twelve thousand men in the course of the afternoon.”[66] When scientific language, with its quantification, its isolation of objects of observation, is applied to something as emotionally charged as Auschwitz, the reader is struck by dissonance.

Levi maps the camp and has a certain idea of the topography of the Lager: “Our Lager is a square of about six hundred yards in length [...] it consists of sixty wooden huts [...].”[67] This is how he reviews twenty-nine blocks, the final one of which is the women’s block, the camp brothel. Once he has completed this review, Levi zooms in on a methodical description of the average block. Here, the place is surveyed drily and unemotionally, in an orderly, methodical, and clear fashion. Dissonance becomes pronounced when Levi describes the parade ground where the daily roll calls were held.[68]

In the camp Levi learns certain objects have functions he could never have guessed in his previous existence. He then *maps these functions*: metal wire can be used to tie boots; feet can be wrapped in rags, and paper can be applied to add a warm layer to clothes. His former map of the world undergoes adjustment and rearrangement under his altered circumstances.

Process Mapping

In Chapter 2, “On the Bottom,” Levi offers a painstaking, sequential, and detailed description of the process every incoming inmate of Auschwitz underwent. This mapping starts with the intimidating wait, next the humiliation of having to strip naked, the shaving of the head, the shower room, getting dressed, the ceremony when new inmates’ names were replaced by serial numbers, arrival at the block, getting to meet the other prisoners as they return from forced labor, roll call, and dispersal. The process is rendered chronologically, one thing leading to the next, in the actual order of events.

In Chapter 8, Levi discusses the camp’s economic system. Using professional terms to produce a *systematic mapping*, he describes the shirt exchange and the people who participated in these “economic” activities: the dealers, thieves, and the exploited inmates, and how this economy was affected by local events. The camp’s internal economy is influenced by the goings-on in the external world. When the tobacco supply in nearby Krakow comes to a temporary standstill, it is felt in the camp in spite of the fence that keeps it isolated from the rest of humanity.[69]

Classification, quantitative reporting, and the various types of mapping are all components of the culture of science supporting Levi in the encounter with trauma and in eventually reproducing it when he struggled to find a rational explanation.[70]

But it is not scientific discipline alone that goes into this work: another dimension too is involved, in which *poetic discipline* plays an important role, namely the formal design, like a metaphor, to help understand reality.[71]

Any writing about the Holocaust must grapple with the paradox of being an attempt to describe what cannot be described, something which leads to the statement that language fails in the face of the actual experience. In *If This Is a Man*, prisoners encounter this incongruency before anything else. There, for the first time, they realized that their language had no words to describe the destruction of a human being. In an instant, with almost prophetic clarity, they understood the harsh reality – they had reached the bottom.[72] Levi's language mirrors this paradox as well as his effort to address it by means of a range of strategies, scientific as well as poetic. His poetic lexicon includes, for instance, metaphoric-analogical structures, Biblical, and mythological allusions. Metaphor, in his writing, does not serve an ornamental purpose. His preferred mode of describing human existence is, as explained below, by conceptual metaphor.

Conceptual Metaphor

In *Metaphors We Live By*,[73] Lakoff and Johnson explain that metaphor, rather than having an ornamental function, is a crucial component in the genesis of conceptual thinking and the cognitive architecture by means of which we make sense of and convey abstract ideas. Referring to intangible, non-concrete experience (like emotions or ideas, time, or death), abstract concepts must be rendered by analogy or other types of reference to concrete perception and experience. Lakoff and Turner argue that the schemata on which conceptual metaphors are based (e.g., life as a journey, life as a stage, life as a flame, death as night, youth as spring) consist of general models that fix typical or prototypical knowledge data into a constant ratio. Data that thus gather under one schema, or alternatively, that branch out from it, are natural subcategories relating to developmental stages, functions, objectives, reasons, results, and so on. The authors identify three groups of conceptual metaphors: conceptual metaphors of orientation, ontological conceptual metaphors, and structural conceptual metaphors.[74]

Conceptual Metaphors of Orientation

This type of metaphor maps a form of spatial orientation – e.g., up-down, inside-outside, foreground-background, center-margins, near-far, surface-depth – onto abstract concepts. Most of our fundamental concepts are organized on the basis of metaphors of orientation. Non-arbitrary, they are grounded in physical reality. Common expressions reflect how often we use this in our everyday life: "He fell ill" or "Cheer up."

Orientation metaphors furnish the domain onto which they are mapped with a spatial aspect. Joy, for instance, will be described in terms of ascent or rising – "high spirits," for instance – and sadness and depression as a falling, descending movement: "Her face fell." These metaphors are based on body experiences: when people are happy, their bodies straighten up, and when they are sad, by contrast, they will contract or hunch. Other concepts in the domain of spatial orientation relate to consciousness and unconsciousness, liberty and enslavement, health, sickness, and death.

In *If This Is a Man*, conceptual metaphors of orientation are notable. From the moment the narrator sets foot in Auschwitz, he reaches for conceptual metaphors as well as ancient mythology as the basic modes of representation for experiences that are beyond words. Even when still en route to the camp, Levi writes that this was a journey towards nothingness, "a journey down there, towards the bottom."[75] The word "bottom," for instance, also appears as the title to Chapter 2, "On the Bottom,"[76] referring both to the mythological narrative concerning the descent into the underworld, as well as to the spatial metaphor for an unsupportable reality.

The predicament of being free or enslaved, too, is expressed by means of the upward/downward orientation, following the same scheme used in the chapter on the Canto of Ulysses. The chapter consists of the episode during which Levi is summoned to clamber out of the dark petrol tank whose bottom he and his comrades have been scrubbing. Levi rises from the depths of the earth towards the sunlight, so as to go out and fetch soup, together with Jean, or "Pikolo," for their group. This momentarily turns into a liberating, cultural outing.[77]

Levi's ideas about humanity are reflected in his use of conceptual metaphors involving rising from the obscure depths towards the light. This type of metaphor reveals a rationalist approach in which human beings struggle against ignorance to gain knowledge and reason. Here we see linguistic and cultural structures reflecting European notions of enlightenment joining together. This rationalist tendency in Levi can be observed in his preference for conceptual metaphors that associate knowledge with fire, light, warmth, awakening, alertness, and ascent.

Structural Conceptual Metaphors

A structural conceptual metaphor maps an abstract concept by means of a narrative structure with a beginning, middle, and end. This allow us to extract aspects from a metaphorical journey narrative, which together offer a mapping of the abstract concept of "life." Here are some such aspects of the analogy between the traveler and the human being passing through her or his life: the continuity and directionality typical of a road and a person's unfolding life; between stations and stages of life; between crossroads and moments of doubt or indecision; between obstacles and difficulties encountered; between real physical goals and life goals; between staying on course and achieving plans; between a turning point and major change, etc. Dante, at the start of the *Divine Comedy*, presents his life in terms of a journey: "In the middle of the journey of our life, I came to/myself in a dark wood, for the straight way was lost."[78] Levi does not merely employ myth as a super-structure that imbues life with tragic meaning. He uses it to map the most basic, universal concepts onto a phenomenon that would appear to defy description. Using metaphor in this way helps him deal with an unknown and unintelligible reality. He tries to explain this incomparably horrible reality to himself by making connections with and transpositions into basic, concrete knowledge.[79] I will discuss Levi's use of the structural conceptual metaphor by considering two metaphors: life as a journey and life as a theater stage.

Life as a Journey

If This Is a Man opens with a journey from Italy to Poland, and the first chapter is, in fact, called "The Journey." In the reality of life in the camp, too, in spite of its clamp-down on movement, the journey becomes an important element. The march to work and back from it, or the hauling of heavy loads along shorter stretches, becomes a concrete metaphor of existence. This existence is cyclic.[80] It is a circular structure which only breaks toward the forward-looking end of the book, leading into freedom.

Life as a Theater Stage

The "stage" as a conceptual metaphor not only constitutes the deep structure of experience but also offers a reflective perspective to both author and reader who take the position, as it were, of spectators at a theater play: "Now the second act begins. Four men with razors, soap-brushes and clippers burst in"[81]; "We seem to be watching some mad play, one of those plays in which the witches, the Holy Spirit and the devil appear"[82]; "But now it is time to stop, it is all over now. This is the last act: the winter has begun, and with it our last battle"[83] This type of dissociation produces restrained representation of the charged reality and creates a distance from which things can be observed from a controlled, even slightly alienated perspective.

Mythology as Metaphor

Mythology, fundamentally, behaves like conceptual metaphor. Myth is a type of narrative that connects abstract and concrete thinking, creating communication among the mental, intellectual, and perceptual domains. This is a natural and familiar function of the brain, and its subtlest expressions can be found in philosophy and poetry. Thus, for example, when Camus wants to illustrate the absurdity of human existence, he uses the myth of Sisyphus, the rock, and the netherworld.[84]

If This Is a Man includes a great deal of mythic material, taken from both the Bible and Greek mythology. The archaic serpent, the Tower of Babel, and the exodus from Egypt are all instances of the first type of reference.[85] An example from Greek mythology is the story of Tantalus. They dream of eating food. They don't only see the food but also feel it in their hands, so concrete. But every time a different circumstance intervenes to prevent the consummation of the act.[86] In telling about the chemistry test, Levi turns to the moment when Oedipus faces the Sphinx: "Alex is briefly dismissed and put aside, and I feel like Oedipus in front of the Sphinx [...]."[87] When he discusses debilitating forced labor, he hints at Sisyphus – for instance, when he describes the hard work of unloading iron pipes, lifting them, and then carrying them to the factory as actual torture.

While for Levi Auschwitz was a reality situated in space and time, it also constituted what he called the "other side," a phenomenon radically exceeding familiar temporal and spatial categories and therefore requiring mythological language. Thus, mythology serves as a *hypo-text*, to structure and conceptualize this impossible reality described in the *hypertext*.[88]

The Myth of the Descent into the Underworld: This is the myth Levi chose as his main hypo-text in *If This Is a Man*. Levi's main source is the "Inferno" from Dante's *Divine Comedy*,[89] a foundational text for every educated Italian. Levi recalls and quotes various passages from this Christian medieval version of hell to portray actual life in Auschwitz: "Auschwitz: a name without significance for us at that time, but it at least implied some place on this earth."[90] Once on "the other side," mythological language is required to "map" concrete reality.

The chapter is called "On the Bottom," and it echoes the underworld, the inferno. The German soldier in Levi's narrative is called Charon, after the man in charge of ferrying the souls of the dead to the underworld of Hades. From this point on, the *Divine Comedy*'s version of the descent into hell becomes the meta-structure for the entire book: "Here I am, then, on the bottom."[91] A separate chapter, "The Canto of Ulysses," which refers crucially to the 26th canto of the Inferno, describing Ulysses in the eighth circle of hell, relies most fully on this material.

The mythic descent into the underworld is a universal trope for a journey of initiation in which the protagonist or hero undergoes processes of identity building.[92] These processes, one cultural expression of which is rites of passage, involve essential stages in the development of personality. Rites of passage, Van Gennep argued, are marked by three stages of initiation: (1) farewell to childhood and passage into adulthood – the stage of separation; (2) move into a transitional, liminal zone; spatially this is represented by a forest, desert, or underworld; this unfamiliar, unusual domain signifies "otherness" (one example is Odysseus' descent into hell); (3) return to civilization and reunification, which is also a move to a new condition, a new understanding of reality. Sometimes this process is presented as rebirth and the acquisition of a new personality, which may even involve an act of re-naming.

To these three stages, I would like to add another one, specific to the artist-as-hero: the formation of culture in response to our awareness of death. This hero can recount, or sing, or set to music his or her encounter with death. Thus, Orpheus looked at death and paid the price of losing his beloved Eurydice in order then to tell her story and that of the underworld in the world of the living, playing his lyre.

All myths referring to the descent into the underworld share their hero's desire to cross the border between life and death to examine the limits of human existence. Though Levi's voyage to hell was forced upon him, his description of Auschwitz – the stages he experienced, his feelings, insights, and responses – all echo the foundational myth about hell. While we have no way of knowing to what extent Levi was familiar with other ancient texts involving similar subject matter – like Sumerian or Akkadian myth – they reflect similar feelings to the traumatic experiences he described. Deeply familiar with Dante's text, unsurprisingly Levi turned to its imagery.

Into the Liminal Zone – Shedding Personal Identity

In the Sumerian myth, Inanna, queen of heaven, goes down into the underworld, on her own initiative – challenging death and seeking to gain control over it.[93] Before setting out on her journey, Inanna dons all the symbols of her divinity. When she arrives in hell, its gates close behind her, as the doors to the palace of death slowly open. Each time a door opens she is forced to take off another garment; and each time she is asked to remove another attribute of her divine status. This gradual humbling and denudation represent the erasure of identity – in this case, Inanna's divine identity. It is death's great power that it can force this exposure. A similar sense of loss of identity through enforced removal of clothes can be found back in Levi's account:

> The door is opened and an SS man enters [...] then we have to undress and make a bundle of the clothes [...]. Finally, another door is opened: here we are, locked in, naked, sheared and standing with our feet in water. [...] we do not dare lift our eyes to look at one another [...].[94]

Authentic Contact with and Reconstitution of the Self

Inanna's descent into the underworld is a rite of passage. Though it connotes a struggle with death, this descent also suggests rebirth. In the case of Odysseus too, hell is a peak experience on his journey home. The descent into hell in Homer's Odyssey Book 11,[95] is a journey to the ultimate "elsewhere" – while at the same time being the highlight of Odysseus' self-formation. From the journey to hell, and his dialogue with the dead, Odysseus gains knowledge that is vital to his development and ensures the success of his journey of initiation. Auschwitz, in Levi's story, served as a kind of a university.[96]

The gradual undoing of the hero's identity takes him to his true essence. It is no coincidence that when the first humans leave Paradise, they cover themselves, while in the narrative of the underworld, people shed their clothes. Cultural coverings are removed on the way to reaching the authentic self. It is paradoxically from the underworld, from the experience of the deeply "other," that these people describe their trauma as the most authentic contact with themselves.

Another element in the myth of the descent into the underworld relevant to Levi's text is the price paid for the ascent back from it. The most dangerous journey, in this kind of experience – the way back home, to civilization, to safety and familiarity – involves great terror. Reaching the desired conclusion takes tactics and effort. So, for instance, Odysseus, on returning home, pretends he is a beggar. Only slowly and carefully does he reveal his identity to his old acquaintances. The end of that particular epic is overshadowed by the story of the destructive return home of Agamemnon. Levi, in *If This Is a Man*, has a recurrent nightmare: in it he attempts to tell visitors about the things that happened to him, but they do not want to hear.

The Cost of Returning from Hell

Another element in the mythology around the descent into the underworld, relevant in Levi's case as well, is the sense that there is no way out of hell without paying a price. Balance must be preserved: when one person exits the underworld, another must take their place:

> Are you ashamed because you are alive in the place of another? [...] You cannot block out such feelings [...] that each one of us (but this time I say "us" in a much vaster, indeed, universal sense) has usurped his neighbor's place and lived in his stead.[97]

This echoes the myth about Inanna's descent into hell. The laws of hell stipulate that the one way in which she can escape death is to supply hell with a human replacement of herself.[98]

The sense of guilt of the survivor who returned from the death camps is quite explicit in Levi's poetry, as I will consider below.

Reconstructing the Culture

Orpheus, the greatest of poets, went down into the underworld to bring Eurydice back to life. He succeeds in convincing Hades, ruler of the underworld, to release Eurydice on condition that he, Orpheus, will not look back at her on their way out of the underworld. But just before they emerge, Orpheus does look back, and Eurydice vanishes, this time forever. Orpheus returns alone to the world of the living. There he immortalizes his love for Eurydice in poetry and music. Orpheus' gaze at the underworld is reminiscent of Levi's work. This is how he reconstitutes his destroyed culture.

In sum, even though, unlike in the original myth, Levi's voyage to hell was not undertaken by his own choice, his description of Auschwitz carries the nucleus myth about hell: He is stripped of all signs of identity; he describes moments of making authentic contact with self-identity; he renders the unabating guilt with which those who survived at the expense of others are tormented, ending with the obsessive need to tell their tale in an attempt to re-constitute culture. Levi tells the story of a man who crossed into the zone of death, looked death in the eye, returned to tell the tale, and withdrew for good.

The Rational Drive in "The Canto of Ulysses"

Levi's chapter "The Canto of Ulysses" in *If This Is a Man* reflects Canto 26 of Dante's "Inferno" in *The Divine Comedy*.[99] In this chapter, Primo Levi emerges from an underground petrol tank, which he had to scrape and clean from the inside, after being called by Jean, or *Pikolo*, to help him bring food to their co-workers. Jean, a student from Alsace, asks Levi to teach him Italian. Levi, in response, recites Canto 26, from the "Inferno," which Italians commonly perceive as a core text of humanism. Levi tries to recall lines from the canto. This project of memorization turns out to be a triumph for civilization and culture over barbarism.

In this chapter the myth of the descent into the underworld takes the form of a palimpsest[100]: a many-layered sheet consisting of a number of superimposed texts. The chapter "The Canto of Ulysses" includes, stimulatingly, seven partly occluded layers of reference. The most ancient source is Homer's *Odyssey*. Odysseus, on his initiation journey, on the way to consolidate his identity, visits the underworld. Here he learns about his past from historical figures who are now dead, then returns to the world of the living with renewed vitality. In Virgil's *Aeneid*, Aeneas, the hero, also pays a visit to the underworld, while in Dante's "Inferno," Dante and Virgil take a stroll through hell, while Virgil informs Dante about the circles of hell. A next, fourth layer in Levi's chapter is situated in school, where the young Levi learns by heart Dante's "Canto of Ulysses." The fifth layer is the main narrative, the hypertext, unfolding in Auschwitz, in which Primo Levi, the teacher, and his student Jean-Pikolo are on their way to bring food to their comrades in the underground petrol tank. This scene turns into a recollection and confirmation of the narrator's cultural past.[101] The sixth layer is the time of writing itself, after the war, in which Levi attempts to remember and reconstruct the experience of Auschwitz, while the seventh and final layer represents the reader, who is expected to hold together all these temporal strata. This palimpsestic quality of the text is achieved by means of a splitting of perspectives into prisms through which the text is orchestrated in a restrained manner, while maintaining historical continuity over and beyond the fragmentation and splitting trauma entails.

Poetry and myth, here, are directly interwoven with scientific expression. This split mode of observation – which represents reality through both scientific and poetic literacy – reproduces a multi-faceted reality, replete with a wealth of representation, and has the effect of keeping pain at a controlled distance. This blending is typical of Levi's writing and it is, as we shall see, painfully fragile. I will dwell on the interactions between these two languages, and what is behind the text's restrained balance – as well as its collapse.

In "The Canto of Ulysses" Levi tries to teach Jean, the Frenchman, some Italian. Surprisingly though, he instructs him in the language of culture rather than in the everyday Italian that could be of use in the camp.[102] On their way to fetch the food for their comrades, Levi tries to remember the verses about Ulysses, a text he learned in high school, in Italy. At this stage of Dante and Virgil's journey, they encounter Ulysses in the eighth circle of hell in which dwell the crooks. Ulysses, speaking from the flames, tells Dante about his final journey. When he concludes his story, he is swallowed back by the fire. Ulysses was punished because he shook off the gods' shackles and tried to sail to the end of the world. In the Renaissance, Ulysses was considered a complex figure who both rebelled against the gods and was driven by intellectual curiosity: A figure who tried to breach the constraints of religious faith and put man at the center of experience. These are the words with which he addresses his sailors when they despair – it is a key text of Renaissance humanism: "Consider your sowing: you were not made to live/ like brutes, but to follow virtue and knowledge."[103]

The virtues of rationalism are a theme in Levi's work. It is his vital source. A detailed analysis of what Levi does and does not recall of the canto, reveals the rational drive underlying his recollection. What does Levi remember of the underlying source the hypo-text? As we shall see, he remembers what will give him strength: the powers of reason which drive him to seek for knowledge.[104]

Canto 26: The Hypo-Text

Dante is eager to know how Ulysses died. Neither Homer, nor Virgil nor Statius mention his death. In Homer's narrative, Odysseus returns home to Attica after his peregrinations, and this is where the story takes leave of him, surrounded by his family. What we are told in the second half of Canto 26 must have been Dante's own invention. His Ulysses tells us about the thirst for knowledge, a desire which seems universal and heroic. This hero will be held back neither by love for his son Telemachus, nor by respect for his old father Laertes, nor even by love of his wife Penelope. His burning desire, his passion to find out about what is beyond what he already knows, translates into an image of Ulysses being caught in flames, which encircle and occlude him.[105] Dante's Ulysses, instead of turning back to Attica, directs his ship to the open sea. He and the small band of his men pass Spain, Morocco, Sardinia, and, finally, the Pillars of Hercules – i.e., the Straits of Gibraltar – then considered the furthest frontier of the inhabited world.

Five months into their journey, Ulysses and his men saw a dark mountain in the distance. Their initial joy quickly turned into tears. The storm wound around their vessel three times, drowning all the sailors "until the sea had closed over us."[106] The tragedy of the shipwreck is outdone by the tragedy that visits Ulysses, an adventurer in search of knowledge beyond anything the human eye had ever witnessed. While his thirst for knowledge turned him into a heroic figure, Ulysses was destined to be punished for his hubris. Dante enacts the role of Ulysses in this canto: He wishes to know about life in the other world. Ulysses' desire to know surpasses his love for his family and his sense of duty toward his men and his city.

What is Ulysses' sin? In the Christian view, it is the fact that he ignores the limits of human knowledge: humility and modesty are of greater importance than knowledge. Even though Dante greatly admires Ulysses, he adopts the orthodox stance and takes a critical view of the intellect's appetite for knowledge. He reminds us that man is not in command of the world: God's unknowable will govern all. Ulysses paid for his curiosity with his life. During his final journey, Ulysses transgressed. He dared to cross the gods' limit. His sin is the sin of seeking to gain knowledge for its own sake, without good measure. Wrapped in eternal flames, Ulysses' soul is isolated from all that surrounds him.

In contrast with Dante's complex and ambivalent criticism, which hesitates between the theological and the rational approaches, between forging out ahead and restraint, scholars of Levi's time saw Ulysses as a secular, Enlightenment hero. This is a human hero, no longer tied up by a transcendental prohibition.

In Homer's foundational text, the story describes Odysseus' adventures as he travels home to his wife Penelope. In his *Divine Comedy*, Dante transforms this original journey into the tale of a catastrophe which is the outcome of hubris.

Though the hero drowns in the attempt to attain an ill-guided goal, in doing so he becomes a symbol of Renaissance man whose insatiable hunger for knowledge sets him apart from the rest of creatures.

The Hypo-Text: What Does Levi Recall?

Hypo-text and hypertext entertain complicated relations. Levi cannot be compared only to Ulysses returning home. His story is also, and mainly, associated with Ulysses burning in hell. Levi adopts Dante's mythological construal of Ulysses, who, wrapped in fire, is only allowed a break to tell the story about his and his fellow soldiers' death. Recollecting this text in the concentration camp, however, gives Levi the strength to survive – it is thanks to this moment of grace that he regains faith in reason.

Levi's chapter opens in the deepest recesses of the earth where six prisoners are working in almost utter darkness. Jean, who needs help with fetching food, asks Levi to come along and leave the petrol tank. This move out of the dark and into the light functions as a metaphor for the shift from ignorance to knowledge; the ascent from the tank up and out denotes the transition from slavery to freedom, a moment of redemption. Primo and Jean, on their way to getting the food, assume the roles of Dante and Virgil.[107] His own choice of Ulysses puzzles Levi: "... The canto of Ulysses. Who knows how or why it comes into my mind."[108] He begins with the passage in which Ulysses, trapped in the flames, struggles to tell his story. It takes a great effort to produce a sound. Levi too has his difficulties: First, he has a hard time translating the passage into reasonably good French, and next he cannot quite recollect the text. He has only limited time to tell the story: as long as it takes them to collect the soup and take it back to the petrol tank. The story, however, says Jagendorf, will not exist if it will not be remembered. About forty years later, in *The Drowned and the Saved*, discussing the intellectual in Auschwitz, Levi will consider how he felt then, struggling to remember. He truly would have offered bread and soup – his very lifeblood – in order to rescue those memories from oblivion. For him, they were essential in restoring a connection to the past, preserving it from being forgotten, and in doing so, strengthening his sense of identity and enabling him to rediscover himself.[109]

What Levi Managed to Remember and Save in Recollecting Ulysses' Words?

Levi might have, unconsciously, sought to appropriate Ulysses' sense of spiritual liberation preceding the catastrophe, in contrast to his own, present physical enslavement. Levi extracted from the episode the very courage that helped Ulysses to overcome his obstacles, as well as the power to survive through one's non-bestial qualities, the ones that define a person as a rational creature even in their darkest hour. He seems to have found the broken link in the chain of culture and to regain his humanity.

Levi experiences a kind of revelation, an epiphany, as his knowledge about the world and about himself changes. His knowledge is no longer casual: he experiences an intimate, private appropriation in which subjective experience transforms into a sublime moment of self-oblivion. It is a profound experience, nothing like that of a high school student who commits poetry to memory. This insight about reason and the freedom it holds for mankind, regardless of place and time, occurs when he and Jean toil most strenuously, carrying the poles on which the soup is transported. Levi urgently needs to share his exceptional experience with Jean:

> Here, listen, Pikolo, open your ears and your mind, you have to understand, for my sake: 'Think of your breed; for brutish ignorance/ Your mettle was not made; you were made men./ To follow after knowledge and excellence.' As if I also was hearing it for the first time: like the blast of a trumpet. Like the voice of God. For a moment I forget who I am and where I am.[110]

This moment is for him a moment of the sublime. Through the Canto of Ulysses, he makes contact with his own free will, an experience of liberation and redemption in the extermination camp. Paradoxically, exactly at the moment when he forgets himself, he makes contact with his true self. Moved by the injunction to be followers of worth and knowledge it is as if, here and now, he had touched something precious. This becomes his rational mission in the world for the rest of his life. Ulysses was the model from which Levi took mental endurance: through willpower and the investigation of existence he became fully human, even if this meant that he might pay with his life. In the camp, what enabled Levi to maintain his sanity was to find a hold in his rational insights.

Levi becomes intensely aware of his obligation to remain a rational person, and of his responsibility for sharing this awareness with others. Once they arrive at the place where he and Pikolo collect the soup, the sublime moment passes, and, much like in the story of Ulysses, the ship, overwhelmed by greater forces, sinks. Again, they find themselves immersed in the camp's passive humiliation, symbolized by the soup.[111]

Between Hypo-Text and Hypertext

Dante's Ulysses, the hero of the hypo-text, is a heroic figure who is entangled in hubris. There are reason and meaning to Dante's hell. The obvious analogy also ironically underlines the differences: Unlike Ulysses, Levi has done nothing to deserve his sojourn in hell. He has not even shown an excessive desire for knowledge. He has fallen victim to the meaningless cruelty of the camp, of which the soup is its symbol.

Finding himself in an actual inferno, Levi draws spiritual sustenance from a fictional analogy, grounded in a theology that allows for cleansing and redemption. The discrepancy raises some questions:

In the deranged reality of the concentration camp, Levi found support in Dante's text as a poem praising reason and knowledge. Unlike Dante, his sojourn in hell was due to no fault of his own. But did the poem continue to offer Levi moral support later in life, after liberation, when needing to process his trauma? Why did Levi ignore contextual differences? What unconscious information surfaced as a result of the comparison? What can we learn from Levi's choice of Ulysses as his paradigm, both in regards of his experience in the camp, and later, in the years to follow? Could this be a form of acting out, with Levi getting addicted to the power of human reason, and extolling it without realizing the price this glorification of knowledge exacted? Is such an adamant pursuit of reason the solution to the afflictions of the camp? Does it offer an answer to the human atrocities to which Levi fell victim? The answer at the end of this chapter is the confusion of languages among the miserable masses, which brings up short Levi's sense of inner elation, confronting it with the camp's traumatic reality. The chapter ends with Dante's words: "until the sea had closed over us."[112]

Avoidance

While Levi's work is consistently dominated by a rational approach, it also reveals, no less powerfully, a quietly subversive strain. This component is characterized by avoidance of contact with the feelings inevitably stirred by traumatic experience. In approaching Levi's writings with a view to these matters I identified the indirect, covert emotional elements I discuss below. Before doing so however, let me first consider some moments when avoidance of contact with the emotions characterizes his textual strategy. I will then outline the more implicit ways in which emotional intensities transform in his texts, especially towards the end of Levi's life. Finally, I will present the traumatic core itself, as we can uniquely glimpse it at the end of Levi's *The Truce*.[113]

What Is Forgotten in "The Canto of Ulysses"

Throughout his life Levi maintained a strong need to discipline his experience, refusing to recognize the reverse need to express the intensity of his feelings regarding chaos, trauma and death. Levi seemed neither to indulge in feelings of guilt, shame or hate, nor to process them. He explained he had consciously adopted aloofness, the transparent sober language of the witness. He wouldn't let himself "weep in the desert."[114]

When we carefully consider what Levi remembered in reciting the canto and what he omitted, his rationalism is, as mentioned, most conspicuous. Levi remembered the verses that convey this message, especially its most famous passage: "Consider your sowing: you were not made to live/ like brutes, but to follow virtue and knowledge."[115] Other things however he forgot, no matter how desperately he tried to retrieve them. Those forgotten verses drew my special attention.[116] Levi did not remember Ulysses' fondness for his son Telemachus; or the ship's voyage and the specific places it visited; or the description of the stars at night, and the travelers' emotional reaction when mount Purgatory came into view. Approaching Purgatory, Ulysses and his comrades are awestruck and full of joy. Soon however, their happiness turns into tears: they are caught up in a storm and drown in the waves: "We rejoiced, but it quickly turned to weeping; for/ from the new land a whirlwind was born and struck/ the forequarter of the ship."[117] What is also missing is a description of the traumatic core: The impact of the gale, the origin of trauma, the source of calamity – all of these have dropped out of his memory, and what remains is only the outcome: "until the sea had closed over us."[118]

To emphasize Ulysses' freedom, Levi several times repeated the journey's "open sea" (*mare aperto*).[119] That he omitted the verse about Ulysses' feelings – joy followed by tears – represents an important aspect of Levi's writing. At this point he did not allow the chaotic elements of his psyche to articulate themselves: they were fragmenting and uncontrollable forces. Throughout his life, arguably, he remained dedicated to imposing order allowing almost no entry to any opposite mental dynamic, of the kind that would give vent to emotional feelings about trauma and death. In April 1981, in his early 60s, Levi wrote the poem "Unfinished Business" in which he mentions everything he regrets not having done. This is how he ends the poem:

> Above all, dear sir, I had in mind/ A marvelous book that would have/ Revealed innumerable secrets, / Alleviated pain and fear,/ Dissolved doubt, given to many people/ The boon of tears and laughter/ You'll find the outline in my drawer,/ In back, with the unfinished business/ I haven't had time to see it through. Too bad./ It would have been a fundamental work.[120]

These lines show how Levi himself felt about stowing his feelings deeply away and leaving them unprocessed: "innumerable secrets [...] tears and laughter [...] in back with the unfinished business [...]" They supply the words of Ulysses' canto Levi did not manage to recollect, "We rejoiced, but it quickly turned to weeping" which described his joy at seeing mount Purgatory and his sadness at not being able to enter it.

Traces of Repressed Feelings

To see whether human reason has the power to control the centaur's drives and passions for any length of time, let's take another look at the story "Quaestio De Centauris." The narrator hoped that the human reason with which the hybrid creature, half human half horse, was endowed could help it live in harmony with its passions. But the encounter with cruel reality leads to a loss of all rational restraint, dooming the centaur to perdition. Levi himself, it seems, kept tight hold of reason's reins for fear of this type of loss, of the crumbling of rational barriers and a release of emotions that might result in the kind of chaos that scared him throughout his life. What is unusual about the story "Quaestio De Centauris" is that it describes a Titanic outburst of love, that leads to destruction and disaster.

Levi only rarely referred to the victim's feelings of terror and shame. One such exceptional occasion is in *The Truce*: Early in the book he mentions a feeling shared by both the liberators and liberated: shame. The four young Russian soldiers who were the first to enter Auschwitz fell silent together with the survivors.[121] The other moments when Levi makes contact with feeling occur on his way back home, with the recognition of the pain of loss, loneliness and the close existence of death. At the very moment when all danger appeared to fade and hope became possible, he was suddenly overwhelmed – as if a dam had broken – by a deeper, more profound sorrow. This pain, long suppressed and pushed to the edges of his awareness by more urgent suffering, now surfaced: the anguish of exile, the ache for the distant home, the weight of loneliness, the loss of friends and youth, and the haunting presence of countless corpses all around him.[122]

When he spends time at the Ka-Be because he is ill and cannot participate in the usual hard labor, or when he is on his way home, after liberation, to his old life in Turin, passing through foreign lands in which he has never set foot, Levi allows for a brief glance at his personal distress. These feelings will not surface again until *The Drowned and the Saved*, written a year before his death. The passage cited from *The Truce*, recounts Levi's personal Odyssey; the title of this book is unsurprising: it is at this point outside time and space that he allows himself access to these deepest emotional strata.

One of the most moving passages in his whole oeuvre appears here, at the end of this book: it is a recurrent dream. Having dropped all his defenses, Levi reveals two dreams, which collapse into one. In the end only one thing defines his identity: the camp's morning call, "Wstawać."[123]

Emotional Traces in Levi's Poetry

Levi, most of whose writing is restrained and controlled, dropped some defenses in his poetry. He wrote poetry only incidentally, but when he did so he exposed different strata. His *Collected Poems* (*Ad Ora Incerta*) was published in 1984.[124] To a correspondent in Switzerland he wrote that the writing of poetry brought into play mental processes he neither understood nor controlled. His rational side, he explained, repressed everything else. As mentioned before, he set great store by being clear. He neither knew nor tried to explain to himself what was concealed behind reason.[125] Levi also described his need to write poetry as a sickness: "every now and then I get this curious infection, like an exanthematic illness that gives you a rash."[126] Increasingly his poetry was dominated by darkness and death. His poems held a sense of despair and opened a window on a different inner world. Some of these poems express an anger and hatred absent from his other work.

In his poetry Levi gave vent to the pain and loneliness which he kept out of his prose. Obsessive survivor's guilt haunts him. In the poem "The Survivor1" he writes: "[…] Go away. I haven't dispossessed anyone,/ Haven't usurped anyone's bread,/ No one died in my place. No one. / Go back into your mist./ It's not my fault if I live and breathe/."[127] Levi turns directly to the spirits of the dead who won't leave him alone, and begs them to go back to their haze. His guilt echoes the earlier mentioned ancient Babylonian myth about Inanna's descent into the underworld, a journey from which no one returns without paying a price. If one wants to escape that place, he or she must find someone else to replace her or him.[128] Maybe the myth points at the source of survivor guilt. Levi puts it unambiguously in an interview with Marco Vigevani: "It is the feeling of being alive in someone else's stead."[129]

Levi's poem "Almanac"[130] reflects fear of the desert, something he also mentioned in his article "On Obscure Writing."[131] The desert symbolized for him the tyranny of the irrational and the breakdown of language, leaving the human being with nothing but a wail. On November 24, 1986, only a few months before his death, Levi published the poem "The Dromedary"[132] in which this extremely threatening desert takes over. The poem offers an ironic description of the advantages of the dromedary, king of the desert. It concludes with a painful reference to the boundless waste of the camel's kingdom: "Yes, I am a servant, but the desert is mine;/ There's no servant without his own kingdom. / Mine is desolation. / It is limitless."[133] Having struggled for a positivist grasp of the world, Levi here admits he belongs in the desert, lacking substance and form, a boundless waste.

Textual Traces of Repressed Feeling: Translating *The Trial* into Italian

A further instance of how the repressed forces of Levi's emotional chaos found a way out is Levi's translation of Kafka's *The Trial*. In 1982, Giuliano Einaudi, Levi's publisher, started a project of new translations by Italian authors of European classics. He offered Conrad's *Lord Jim* to Italo Calvino and Flaubert's *Madame Bovary* to Natalia Ginzburg. To Levi, he turned with Kafka's *The Trial*. Though Levi accepted the offer, the task was burdensome and the result unremarkable. When the book came out in 1983, Levi wrote that something about Kafka's writing intimidated him and when translating the novel, he was aware of his own defensiveness. His own writing, by contrast, was grounded in logical and orderly thinking. He had not gone Kafka's way. Kafka had never been one of his favorite authors. He felt attacked by the *Trial* as soon as he began translating it and felt he had to defend himself. He had never chosen Kafka's way – giving free rein to what lies "down Below" in his subconscious.[134] Contact with the irrational, so it would seem, made Levi sick. This intense reaction is a kind of acting-out in relation to the emotional topic, and it testifies to a solid defense mechanism constructed against contact with the unconscious, uncontrolled irrational, whether in his translation work on Kafka or in his own poetry.

Suicide: A Case of Acting Out?

In the chapter on the intellectual in Auschwitz, in *The Drowned and the Saved*, the extermination camp is presented as a totally evacuating experience. Still, at the end of the chapter, Levi sticks to his motivation to live and fend off death. He never devoted himself to death. As he testified, he had many other things to keep himself busy, like finding bread, avoiding hard work or interpreting the signs and faces around him. The aims of life in the Lager, he contended, were the best defense against death.[135]

Throughout his life he had done everything to fend it off. But perhaps in time death slowly made its way into his life; the energy he had put into repressing it ran out, leaving him face to face with the thing he had always avoided.

Late in 1986 Levi suffered another bout of depression. It was compounded by the fact that he was in charge of looking after both his ailing mother and mother-in-law.[136] Two TV interviews from that time reveal how serious his condition was. He felt he had nothing more to say.[137] To his English translator, Ruth Feldman, he wrote he was going through the worst period in his life – worse than Auschwitz because being no longer young, there was nothing left to hold on to.[138] On February 7, 1987 he wrote to his friend David Mendel, a British physician, that he was suffering from deep depression, had lost all interest in writing and even in reading, that he felt weak and did not want to meet anyone, not a psychiatrist either.[139]

In an interview he gave shortly before his death to Roberto Di Caro, he was more exposed than ever.[140] He said he was surprised that he had been able to write *If This Is a Man*, *The Truce*, *Natural Histories*, and part of *The Periodic Table* while still working as a chemist, while now that he was no longer employed, he was both writing less and with less intensity. Then he added:

> The truth is I am living a neurotic life, with draining gaps between one book and the next; [...] every now and then, I have the impression that the cupboard is bare, that I have nothing more to say, no more stories to tell [...] I'm not very balanced at all. I go through long periods of imbalance, no doubt linked to my concentration-camp experience. I find it very hard to cope with problems. This side of myself I've never written about [...] I am not a strong man. Not at all.[141]

Levi observed the discrepancy between his writing and his actual life:

> In my books [...] I see [...] an immense need to put things in order, to put order back into a world of chaos, to explain to myself and to others. On a day-to-day basis, however, my life is very different, unfortunately it is much less methodological and systematic. Writing is a way of creating order.[142]

These words disclose Levi's paradoxical character: Two forces in constant struggle, with only one of them, the voice of reason, gaining public expression. The other voice, associated with fragmentation, the irrational voice which was not so balanced – this voice was quite silenced, repressed. Wanting out, this voice eventually, might pointing him to his death.

On Saturday morning April 11, 1987, four days before Jewish Passover, Italian television announced that Primo Levi had fallen to his death from the stairs of his third-floor apartment. He had left no message or letter, and the autopsy revealed no signs of violence. Two days later he was buried at Turin's Jewish cemetery. His tombstone carries his name, his concentration camp number, 174517, the dates of his birth and death.[143]

In the story "The Bridge,"[144] Levi describes the collapse of a bridge. slowly, piece by piece, almost as if it were in pain or trying to resist. This struck him with the same sorrow one feels at a person's death. Naturally, when someone dies or a structure falls, says Levi, there must be a reason, perhaps even not a single one, and even if there is, it may remain unknowable. Still, he reminded himself and may be also us, the readers, it was too soon to draw conclusions.[145]

These words qualify anything I might have suggested by way of one clear explanation of Levi's suicide. Yet we cannot reflect on his death, and the light it cast on his life, without taking the option of suicide into account.

The obvious assumption is that Auschwitz belatedly took another life, or as Eli Wiesel put it: "Primo Levi died at Auschwitz forty years later."[146] Others associated his death with the deaths of other intellectuals, like Paul Celan, Jean Améry, and Bruno Bettelheim, who killed themselves many years after returning from the extermination camps. In a last interview before he committed suicide in 1990, Bruno Bettelheim, who had survived Dachau and Buchenwald, said that survivors of these places had only ostensibly survived. He believed that this was why people like Primo Levi ended their own lives because within them the terror of the concentration camps was ever present. He argued that for those who were in the camps it was as if they "always lived on the barbed wire."[147]

Whether it is accompanied by a final note or not, the act of suicide remains a mystery. Cynthia Ozick read *The Drowned and the Saved* as a suicide note.[148] Levi, wrote Ozick, was known for his optimism, his un-angry and nonviolent approach, the absence of any apparent drive for revenge. He did not voice accusations, loud complaints and outcries. When many other writers were explicit about questions of guilt and forgiveness, he suppressed such issues. His way was to describe things – painstakingly, analytically, transparently. Ozick believed, however, that *The Drowned and the Saved* reveals a change in tone. While it begins almost tepidly and calmly, it grows slowly toward something explosive. Such is the buildup of pressure and rage that, in the final chapter, avoidance gives way to an emotional hurricane. From the final pages of the book, everything that has hitherto been held back now erupts. She reads the book as of "blows returned by a pen on fire."[149]

The Drowned and the Saved, argues Ozick, comes to close a decades-long gap of avoidance, with forces which, having been in abeyance throughout, erupting in the author's final work.

So, it seems that Levi spent his entire life trying to by-pass his unconscious, by keeping the rational and irrational, the conceptual and pre-conceptual, reason and the drives, carefully separate. This exclusion and dread of his emotional experience, I believe, contributed to the emergence of cracks in his personality, which then, with the passing of time, may have led to the inevitable end. Much like in his "Quaestio de Centauris," Levi did not manage to forge a link between the emotions – which he so strenuously tried to restrain – and the rational. When, in the end, his emotions broke loose from reason's tight hold, this might have led to his end.

The Orphic Gaze: An Eye-Witness Account

One chemical element conspicuously absent from Levi's *The Periodic Table* is oxygen – the element we need to breathe. Doesn't this suggest an ongoing process of (mental) suffocation or drowning – to which the title of *The Drowned and the Saved* refers? The word "drowned" – *sommersi* in Italian – derives from a line in Dante's "Inferno" which refers to those in the fifth circle, who are drowning in their own tears: "[…] I must make verses/ […] for the twentieth song/ […] which is of those submerged (ch'e d'I sommersi)./ I was already bent over to gaze into the/ uncovered depth which was bathed with anguished/ weeping";[150] Levi's testimony carries the imprint of the witness who, having been saved from the storm, is accompanied for the remainder of his life by the experience of drowning. This Orphic perspective, acquired by one who has witnessed hell and now, restored to the world, represents it in the form of a poetic narrative, reflects the dividing line between reason and madness, the same line which also separates between the saved and the drowned.

One of the most powerful passages Levi wrote appears in *The Truce*. I have already mentioned it. It describes the arrival in Auschwitz of the four Russian infantry men, the camp's liberators. It is from their eyes, that the victims gather how far gone they are.

Levi's story is that of a person who encounters death and returns to tell what he saw, then to depart again. This is Levi's Orphic gaze. Like Ulysses, Levi too tells his story by emerging from the conflagration – and once he's done with the telling, he will vanish again into the devouring flames. The need to tell the story is obsessive, turning the act of satisfying the need into something therapeutic. Levi said that he felt a need to write and that writing, for him, was tantamount to undergoing psychoanalytic treatment.[151] I already mentioned a dream Levi had during his time in the concentration camp, about returning home to his family, and when telling them what happened, they did not believe him. He described this as tantalizing, like "almost eating," the food never reaching your mouth. The same was true about his need to talk about his experience. At a later stage, writing came to substitute for talking.[152] Telling the story, for Levi, was an act of release fulfilling a function similar to confession for Catholics and psychoanalysis for patients.

In the introduction of *If This Is a Man* Levi mentioned, Levi contest that the idea for writing the book was originated during his time in the camp, driven by a powerful urge to share the experience with others. For him, writing was primarily a means of inner liberation.[153]

In *The Periodic Table*, in the chapter entitled "Chrome," he recounts how by writing the book down he found peace for a while and felt himself a man again.[154]

Speaking out, for one who had experienced such extreme trauma; making himself heard publicly and openly, required a difficult inner struggle. Celan expressed a similar struggle in a line appearing in his poem "The Shofar Place": "hear deep in/ with your mouth."[155] In the course of speaking and writing about the trauma "with your mouth," an inverse action too occurred of listening inward.

As mentioned, *The Drowned and the Saved* opens with a quote from Coleridge's "Ballad of the Ancient Mariner": "Since then, at an uncertain hour,/That agony returns:/And till my ghastly tale is told/This heart within me burns."[156] The sailor asks us, again and again, to hear his testimony. The utterly baffling can be accommodated only once it has been witnessed. Only in this way the testimony is validated.

For Levi, writing about trauma was a controlled way of dealing with it. The attempt to make rational sense of Auschwitz appears a productive effort at processing. In fact, however, it turns out to be a fragile, external cover which failed to hold back irrational, emotional intensities. The need to tell was entailed by the strong urge to gain control while avoiding contact with the underlying threatening feeling.[157]

The various expressions of avoidance I have mentioned may have been the only, partly present traces of acting out, which in turn may have been responsible for Levi's collapse. The "desert" which terrified him so much was looming all along, and when rational defenses failed boundlessness revealed itself. This is when trauma showed its persistent quality, causing the living flesh to tremble – something to which he testified at the end of the novel *The Truce*:

> I am in the Lager once more, and nothing is true outside the Lager. All the rest was a brief pause, a deception of the senses, a dream; my family, nature in flower, my home. Now this inner dream, this dream of peace, is over, and in the outer dream, which continues gelid, a well-known voice resounds: a single word, not imperious, but brief and subdued. It is the dawn command of Auschwitz, a foreign word, feared and expected: get up, "Wstawać."[158]

Notes

1 Roberto Di Caro, *The Essential and the Superfluous in the Voice of Memory*, in *Primo Levi Interviews 1961–1987*, eds. Marco Belpoliti and Robert Gordon (The New York Press, 2001), 169.
2 Myriam Anissimov, *Primo Levi: Tragedy of an Optimist*, trans. Steve Cox (The Overlook Press, 1999).
3 Ferdinando Camon, *Conversations with Primo Levi*, trans. John Shepley (Marlboro Press, 1989), 5–6.
4 Primo Levi, *The Invisible World*, in *Other People's Trades*, trans. Raymond Rosenthal (Summit Books, 1989), 58–62.
5 Levi, *Invisible World*, 58.
6 Anissimov, *Primo Levi: Tragedy of an Optimist*, 31.
7 Anissimov, *Primo Levi: Tragedy of an Optimist*, 30.

8 Primo Levi, *The Drowned and the Saved*, trans. Raymond Rosenthal (Summit Books, 1988), 132.
9 Immanuel Kant, *What Is Enlightenment?* https://www.columbia.edu/acis/ets/CCREAD/etscc/kant.html.
10 Levi, *Drowned and the Saved*, 139.
11 Levi, *Drowned and the Saved*, 141.
12 Primo Levi, *On Obscure Writing*, trans. Raymond Rosenthal, in *Other People's Trades* (Summit Books, 1989), 169–175.
13 Levi, *On Obscure Writing*, 171.
14 Camon, *Conversations*, 21–24.
15 Camon, *Conversations*, 21–24.
16 Levi, *On Obscure Writing*, 171–172.
17 Levi, *Drowned and the Saved*, 97.
18 Primo Levi, *The Periodic Table*, trans. Raymond Rosenthal (Schocken Books, 1984).
19 See below for an elaborate discussion.
20 Immanuel Kant, *Critique of Judgment*, trans. James Creed Meredith (Clarendon Press, 1952), 91.
21 Primo Levi, *If This Is a Man, the Truce*, trans. Stuart Woolf (Sphere, [1958] 1988), 115–121.
22 Jean Améry, *At the Mind's Limits*, trans. Sidney Rosenfeld and Stella P. Rosenfeld (Indiana University Press and the United States Holocaust Memorial Museum, 1980), Kindle, 19
23 Levi, *Drowned and the Saved*, 141–142.
24 Samuel Taylor Coleridge, *The Rime of the Ancient Mariner*, vii (1798), 584–588. https://resources.saylor.org/wwwresources/archived/site/wp-content/uploads/2014/05/ENGL404-Coleridge-The-Rime-of-the-Ancient-Mariner.pdf.
25 Levi, *If This Is a Man.*
26 Primo Levi, Interview with Paolo Spriano, "L'avventura di Primo Levi", *L' Unita*, 14 July 1963, in Anissimov, *Primo Levi*, 294.
27 Mirna Cicioni, *Primo Levi: Bridges of Knowledge* (Berg, 1995), 49–50.
28 Anissimov, *Primo Levi*, 299.
29 Cicioni, *Primo Levi: Bridges of Knowledge.*
30 Primo Levi, *Collected Poems*, trans. Ruth Feldman and Brian Swann (Faber and Faber, 1992).
31 Primo Levi, *The Wrench*, trans. William Weaver (Summit Books, 1987).
32 Primo Levi, *If Not Now, When?*, trans. William Weaver (Summit Books, 1985).
33 Levi, On Obscure Writing.
34 Levi, *Drowned and the Saved.*
35 Primo Levi, *The Mirror Maker*, trans. Raymond Rosenthal (Schocken Books, 1989).
36 Dante Alighieri, *Inferno*, trans. Robert M. Durling (Oxford University Press, [1321], 1996).
37 Cynthia Ozick, *What Henry James Knew, and Other Essays on Writers* (Random House, 1994).
38 Giuseppe Grassano, *A Conversation with Primo Levi*, in Marco Belpoliti and Robert Gordon, eds., *Primo Levi Interviews, 1961–1987* (The New Press, 2001), 126.
39 Edoardo Fadini, "Science Fiction I", in *Primo Levi Interviews, 1961–1987*, eds. Marco Belpoliti and Robert Gordon (The New Press, 2001), 85.
40 See Marco Belpoliti, "I Am a Centaur", in *Primo Levi Interviews*, eds. Marco Belpoliti and Robert Gordon.
41 The Greek, mythological figure of the chimera has the head of a lion, the body of a goat, and a snake's or dragon's tail.

42 Primo Levi, *The Complete Works of Primo Levi, Quaestio de Centauris* in *Natural Histories*, trans. Jenny McPhee (Liveright, 2015), Kindle, 509–521.
43 For a different interpretation of this story as a traumatic representation of Levi's Holocaust experience, both as an individual and as a member of the Italian Jewish community, see Felice Italo Beneduce, "'Io Sono Un Centauro' –Betrayal in Primo Levi's Quaestio De Centauris", *Nemia Italian Studies 32* (2009), 27–61.
44 Marco Belpoliti, "I am a Centaur".
45 Levi, *Quaestio de Centauris*, 509–510.
46 https://www.merriam-webster.com/dictionary/colophon.
47 Tzvetan Todorov, *The Fantastic: A Structural Approach to a Literary Genre*, trans. Richard Howard (Cornell University Press, 1975), 24–33.
48 Levi, *Quaestio de Centauris*, 516.
49 Dina Lucha, "Il suono e la mente", Rai, seconda reta radiofonice, 4.10.1982, in *Convesations and Interviews 1963–1987* (Am Oved, 2007), 51. [Hebrew].
50 Scientific method is based on methodical, empirical observations, quantification, and organization. From this, conclusions are drawn to formulate theories; the questioning or testing of these theories and their re-examination with reference to external reality. Richard Klausner, *National Science Education Standards* (National Academy Press, 1994).
51 Primo Levi and Leonardo De Benedetti, *Auschwitz Report*, trans. Judith Woolf, ed. Robert S.C. Gordon (Verso, [1946] 2015).
52 Karl William, director. France 3 (undated).
53 Roberto Di Caro, *The Essential and the Superfluous*, in Levi, *Conversations and Interviews*, 169.
54 Levi, *If This Is a Man*, 56.
55 Levi, *If This Is a Man*, 57.
56 Levi, *If This Is a Man*, 61.
57 Levi, *If This Is a Man*, 47.
58 Albert Camus, *The Myth of Sisyphus and Other Essays*, trans. Justin O'Brien (Hamilton, [1942] 1955).
59 Levi, *If This Is a Man*, 93.
60 Klausner, *Science Education.*
61 Levi, *The Periodic Table*, 203–204.
62 Levi, *If This Is a Man*, 93–106.
63 Levi, *If This Is a Man*, 93.
64 Levi, *If This Is a Man*, 96.
65 Levi, *If This Is a Man*, 98–106.
66 Levi, *If This Is a Man*, 134.
67 Levi, *If This Is a Man*, 37.
68 Levi, *If This Is a Man*, 39.
69 Levi, *If This Is a Man*, 83–92.
70 Levi, *Periodical Table*, 153.
71 Camon, *Conversations*, 19–20.
72 Levi, *If This Is a Man*, 32.
73 George Lakoff and Mark Johnson, *Metaphors We Live By* (University of Chicago Press, 1980).
74 George Lakoff and Mark Turner, *More Than Cool Reason: A Field Guide to Poetic Metaphor* (Chicago University Press, 1989); Eleanor H. Rosch, "Natural Categories", *Cognitive Psychology 4:3* (1973), 328–350.
75 Levi, *If This Is a Man*, 23.
76 Levi, *If This Is a Man*, 28.
77 Levi, *If This Is a Man*, 115, 117, 118.
78 Alighieri, *Inferno*, 27.

79 Levi, *If This Is a Man*, 121.
80 Levi, *If This Is a Man*, 68.
81 Levi, *If This Is a Man*, 29.
82 Levi, *If This Is a Man*, 31.
83 Levi, *If This Is a Man*, 143.
84 Wallace Fowlie, *A Reading of Dante's Inferno* (Chicago University Press, 1981), 167.
85 Levi, *If This Is a Man*, 44.
86 Levi, *If This Is a Man*, 67.
87 Levi, *If This Is a Man*, 111.
88 A hypertext is a text which relates to a hypo-text, an earlier text in culture. See Gérard Genette, *Palimpsests: Literature in the Second Degree* (University of Nebraska Press, 1997), 5, 398–399.
89 Alighieri, *Divine Comedy*, *Inferno*.
90 Levi, *If This Is a Man*, 23.
91 Levi, *If This Is a Man*, 42.
92 Arnold van Gennep, *The Rites of Passage*, trans. Monika G. Vizedon and Gabrielle L. Caffee (Routledge, 1977).
93 Shin Shifra and Jacob Klein, *In Those Distant Days: Anthology of Mesopotamian Literature* (Am Oved, 2010), 351–367. [Hebrew]. See also the same Akkadian story told about Ishtar descending to the netherworld in B. R. Foster, *Before the Muses. An Anthology of Akkadian Literature* (CDL Press, 2005), 499–504.
94 Levi, *If This Is a Man*, 28–33.
95 Homer, *The Kingdom of Dead*. https://classics.domains.skidmore.edu/lit-campus-only/primary/translations/Homer%20Od%2011.pdf.
96 Levi, *Drowned and the Saved*, 141.
97 Levi, *Drowned and the Saved*, 81–82.
98 Shifra and Klein, *In Those Distant Days: Anthology of Mesopotamian Literature in Hebrew*, p. 362, Line 287–289.
99 Alighieri, *Inferno*, Canto 26, pp. 399–405.
100 A text which has been written on top of an earlier, erased text, usually on papyrus or parchment. At times the previous text can be seen glimmering through.
101 See a very thorough analysis of this chapter by Zvi Jagendorf, "Primo Levi Goes for Soup and Remembers Dante", *Raritan 12:4* (1993), 31–51.
102 Jagendorf, "Primo Levi Goes for Soup and Remembers Dante".
103 Alighieri, *Divine Comedy*, *Inferno*, 405, Canto 26. Lines 118–120.
104 Rina Dudai, "Primo Levi Speaks from the Flames", *Alpayim 25* (2003), 133–154. [Hebrew]; Rina Dudai, "Poetic Language as a Mode of Coping with Holocaust Trauma in Primo Levi's and Aharon Appelfeld's Work", *Mikan 5* (2005), 101–110. [Hebrew]; Uri Cohen, "Consider If This Is a Man: Primo Levi and the Figure of Ulysses", *Jewish Social Studies: History, Culture, Society 18:2* (2012), 40–69.
105 Fowlie, *Reading*, 168.
106 Dante, *Inferno*, 405, Canto 26. Line 142.
107 Jagendorf, *Primo Levi Goes for Soup and Remembers Dante*, 50.
108 Levi, *If This Is a Man*, 118.
109 Levi, *Drowned and the Saved*, 139–140.
110 Levi, *If This Is a Man*, 119.
111 Cicioni, *Primo Levi: Bridges of Knowledge*, 35, 136.
112 Alighieri, *Inferno*, 405, Line 142.
113 Levi, *If This Is a Man*, *The Truce*.
114 Levi, *On Obscure Writing*.
115 Alighieri, *Inferno*, Canto 26, 118–120, 405.
116 Dudai, *Modes of Coping with Trauma in the Holocaust Literature*; Dudai, "Primo Levi"; Dudai, "Poetic Language".

117 Alighieri, *Inferno*, 405, 136–138.
118 Alighieri, *Inferno*, 405, line 142.
119 Alighieri, *Inferno*, 403, line 100.
120 Primo Levi, *Collected Poems. Unfinished Business*, trans. Ruth Feldman and Brian Swann (Faber and Faber, 1992), 47.
121 Levi, *If This Is a Man*, 188–189.
122 Levi, *If This Is a Man*, 190.
123 Levi, *If This Is a Man*, 378.
124 Levi, *Collected Poems.*
125 Anissimov, *Primo Levi*, 320.
126 Giuseppe Grassano in *Primo Levi Interviews*, 132.
127 Primo Levi, *The Survivor.* In *Collected Poems*, 64
128 Shifra and Klein, *In Those Distant Days: Anthology of Mesopotamian Literature in Hebrew*, 362, 287–289.
129 Marco Vigevani, *Words, Memory, Hope.* In Primo Levi Interviews 1961–1987 (The New York Press, 2001), 254.
130 Levi, Almanac, *Collected Poems*, 98.
131 Levi, "On Obscure Writing", 171.
132 Levi, The Dromedary, *Collected Poems*, 97.
133 Levi, The Dromedary, *Collected Poems*, 97.
134 Federico De Melis, *An Assault Called Franz Kafka.* In *Primo Levi Interviews* 1961–1987 (The New York Press, 2001), 156.
135 Levi, *Drowned and the Saved, The Intellectual in Auschwitz*, 148.
136 Cicioni, *Primo Levi: Bridges of Knowledge*, 169.
137 Anissimov, *Primo Levi*, 394.
138 Anissimov, *Primo Levi*, 396.
139 Anissimov, *Primo Levi*, 397–398.
140 Di Caro. *The Essential and the Superfluous.* In *Primo Levi Interviews*, 167–175.
141 Di Caro. *The Essential and the Superfluous.* In *Primo Levi Interviews*, 169–170, 173–174.
142 Di Caro. *The Essential and the Superfluous.* In *Primo Levi Interviews*, 169–170, 173–174.
143 Cicioni, *Primo Levi: Bridges of Knowledge*, 171.
144 Primo Levi, *The Bridge, The Complete Works of Primo Levi* (Liveright, Kindle 2015), 1042–1063.
145 Levi, *The Bridge, The Complete Works of Primo Levi*, 1059–1060.
146 Cicioni, *Primo Levi. Bridges of Knowledge*, 171.
147 Cicioni, *Primo Levi. Bridges of Knowledge*, 171.
148 Cynthia Ozick, "Primo Levi's Suicide Note", in *Metaphor and Memory* (Vintage Books, 1991), 34–48.
149 Ozick, "Primo Levi's Suicide Note", 46.
150 Dante, *Inferno*, Canto 20: 1–6, 305.
151 Camon, *Conversations*, 41–43.
152 Camon, *Conversations*, 41–42.
153 Levi, *If This Is a Man*, 15.
154 Levi, *The Periodic Table*, 151.
155 Celan Paul, *Poems of Paul Celan, The Shofar Place*, trans. John Felstiner (W. W. Norton, 2001), 361.
156 Coleridge, *Rime of the Ancient Mariner*, ll, 582–585.
157 Dudai, *Modes of Coping*; Dudai, "The Poetic Language". Also see, Yochai Ataria, *The Death of the Witness in the Testimony Period, Maarag* (2015), The Magnes Press, 177–214. [Hebrew].
158 Levi, *Truce*, 379–380.

References

Alighieri, Dante, *The Divine Comedy vol. 1 Inferno*, trans. Robert M. Durling (Oxford University Press, [1321] 1996).

Améry, Jean, *At the Mind's Limits*, trans. Sidney Rosenfeld and Stella P. Rosenfeld (Indiana University Press and the United States Holocaust Memorial Museum, 1980), Kindle.

Anissimov, Myriam, *Primo Levi: Tragedy of an Optimist*, trans. Steve Cox (The Overlook Press, 1999).

Ataria, Yochai, *The Death of the Witness in the Testimony Period, Maarag* (2015), Magnes Press, 177–214. [Hebrew].

Belpoliti, Marco, "I Am a Centaur", in Belpoliti Marco and Gordon Robert, eds., *Primo Levi Interviews.*

Belpoliti, Marco and Gordon, Robert, eds., *Primo Levi Interviews 1961–1987* (The New York Press, 2001).

Beneduce, Felice Italo, "'Io Sono Un Centauro' – Betrayal in Primo Levi's Quaestio De Centauris", *Nemia Italian Studies 32* (2009), 27–61.

Camon, Ferdinando, *Conversations with Primo Levi*, trans. John Shepley (Marlboro Press, 1989).

Camus, Albert, *The Myth of Sisyphus and Other Essays*, trans. Justin O'Brien (Hamilton, [1942] 1955).

Celan, Paul, *Poems of Paul Celan, The Shofar Place*, trans. John Felstiner (W. W. Norton, 2001), 361.

Cicioni, Mirna, *Primo Levi: Bridges of Knowledge* (Berg, 1995).

Cohen, Uri, "Consider If This Is a Man: Primo Levi and the Figure of Ulysses", *Jewish Social Studies: History, Culture, Society 18:2* (2012), 40–69.

Coleridge, Samuel Taylor, *The Rime of the Ancient Mariner*, vii (1798), 584–588. https://resources.saylor.org/wwwresources/archived/site/wp-content/uploads/2014/05/ENGL404-Coleridge-The-Rime-of-the-Ancient-Mariner.pdf

Di Caro, Roberto, "The Essential and the Superfluous in the Voice of Memory", in Belpoliti Marco and Gordon Robert, eds., *Primo Levi Interviews 1961–1987* (The New York Press, 2001), 167–175.

De Melis, Federico, *An Assault Called Franz Kafka*. In *Primo Levi Interviews 1961–1987* (The New York Press, 2001), 153–160.

Dudai, Rina. "Modes of Coping with the Trauma in the Holocaust Literature (A. Appelfeld, Ka-Tzetnik, P. Levi. (2000). (Doctoral Thesis, Hebrew University).

Dudai, Rina, "Primo Levi Speaks from the Flames", *Alpayim 25* (2003), 133–154. [Hebrew].

Dudai, Rina, "Poetic Language as a Mode of Coping with Holocaust Trauma in Primo Levi's and Aharon Appelfeld's Work", *Mikan 5* (2005), 101–110. [Hebrew].

Fadini, Edoardo, "Science Fiction I", in Belpoliti Marco and Gordon Robert, eds., *Primo Levi Interviews, 1961–1987* (The New Press, 2001), 84–86.

Foster3, B. R., *Before the Muses. An Anthology of Akkadian Literature* (CDL Press, 2005), 499–504.

Fowlie, Wallace, *A Reading of Dante's Inferno* (Chicago University Press, 1981).

Genette, Gérard, *Palimpsests: Literature in the Second Degree* (University of Nebraska Press, 1997), 5, 398–399.

Grassano, Giuseppe, *A Conversation with Primo Levi*, in Belpoliti Marco and Gordon Robert, eds., *Primo Levi Interviews, 1961–1987* (The New Press, 2001), 121–135.

Homer, *The Kingdom of Dead.* https://classics.domains.skidmore.edu/lit-campus-only/primary/translations/Homer%20Od%2011.pdf

Jagendorf, Zvi, "Primo Levi Goes for Soup and Remembers Dante", *Raritan 12:4* (1993), 31–51.

Kant, Immanuel, *What Is Enlightenment?* https://www.columbia.edu/acis/ets/CCREAD/etscc/kant.html

Kant, Immanuel, *Critique of Judgment*, trans. James Creed Meredith (Clarendon Press, 1952).

Klausner, Richard, *National Science Education Standards* (National Academy Press, 1994).

Lakoff, George and Johnson, Mark, *Metaphors We Live By* (University of Chicago Press, 1980).

Lakoff, George and Turner, Mark, *More Than Cool Reason: A Field Guide to Poetic Metaphor* (Chicago University Press, 1989).

Levi, Primo, *If This Is a Man, the Truce*, trans. Stuart Woolf (Sphere, [1958] 1988).

Levi, Primo, Interview with Paolo Spriano, "L'avventura di Primo Levi", *L' Unita*, 14 July 1963, in Anissimov, *Primo Levi*, 294.

Levi, Primo, *The Periodic Table*, trans. Raymond Rosenthal (Schocken Books, 1984).

Levi, Primo. *If Not Now, When?*, trans. William Weaver (Summit Books, 1985).

Levi, Primo, *The Wrench*, trans. William Weaver (Summit Books, 1987).

Levi, Primo, *The Drowned and the Saved*, trans. Raymond Rosenthal (Summit Books, 1988).

Levi, Primo, *On Obscure Writing*, trans. Raymond Rosenthal, in *Other People's Trades* (Summit Books, 1989), 169–175.

Levi, Primo, *The Invisible World*, in *Other People's Trades*, trans. Raymond Rosenthal (Summit Books, 1989), 58–62.

Levi, Primo, *The Mirror Maker*, trans. Raymond Rosenthal (Schocken Books, 1989).

Levi, Primo, *Collected Poems, trans.* Ruth Feldman and Brian Swann (Faber and Faber, 1992).

Levi, Primo, *The Bridge, the Complete Works of Primo Levi* (Liveright, 2015), Kindle, 1042–1063.

Levi, Primo, *The Complete Works of Primo Levi, Quaestio de Centauris in Natural Histories*, trans. McPhee Jenny (Liveright, 2015), Kindle, 509–521.

Levi, Primo, *Translating Kafka, the Complete Works of Primo Levi* (Liveright, 2015), Kindle, 2349.

Levi, Primo and De Benedetti, Leonardo, *Auschwitz Report*, trans. Judith Woolf, ed. Robert S. C. Gordon (Verso, [1946] 2015).

Lucha, Dina, "Il suono e la mente" Rai, seconda reta radiofonice, 4.10.1982, in *Convesations and Interviews 1963–1987,* trans. Yizchak Garti, ed. Atalia Zilber (Am Oved, 2007), 45–56. [Hebrew].

Ozick, Cynthia, "Primo Levi's Suicide Note", in *Metaphor and Memory* (Vintage Books, 1991), 34–48.

Ozick, Cynthia, *What Henry James Knew, and Other Essays on Writers* (Random House, 1994).

Rosch, Eleanor H., "Natural Categories", *Cognitive Psychology 4:3* (1973), 328–350.

Shifra, Shin and Klein, Jacob, *In Those Distant Days: Anthology of Mesopotamian Literature* (Am Oved, 2010), 351–367. [Hebrew].

Todorov, Tzvetan, *The Fantastic: A Structural Approach to a Literary Genre*, trans. Richard Howard (Cornell University Press, 1975).
van Gennep, Arnold, *The Rites of Passage*, trans. Monika G. Vizedon and Gabrielle L. Caffee (Routledge, 1977).
Vigevani, Marco, *Words, Memory, Hope*. In *Primo Levi Interviews 1961–1987* (The New York Press, 2001), 250–257.
William, Karl, director. France 3 (undated).

Part Three

In Search of a Form for the Primal Scream

Chapter 6

In Search of a Form for the Primal Scream

Discussion and Conclusions

A scream must find its form.[1]

I was left with a sense of suffocation when I put down Aharon Appelfeld's *Searing Light* (1980). A heavy, wordless anguish took hold of me: What was it about this text that left me feeling like this?

The more I dwelled on the text, the clearer it became that my reaction was prompted by the book's traces of traumatic events. I felt "lost in the fog," as Sebald once put it when describing how the reader proceeds with the text after the earlier-mentioned traumatic subject disappeared from view.[2] In its restrained way, Appelfeld's text describes the difficulties experienced by some adolescent boys, Holocaust survivors, who immigrate to Israel at the time of the state's foundation. The clash between the narrative's restraint and its subdued almost invisible subject, on the one hand, and the charged experience the text embodies, on the other, became a formative experience in my work on Appelfeld's writing.

Restraint is generally considered a hallmark of Appelfeld's style. As I mentioned before, the judges, when Appelfeld received the prestigious Israel Prize in 1983, emphasized Appelfeld's unique approach, having succeeded to give form to the human condition in a restrained, subtle, and elegant style. The critics often return to these two aspects of his writing: restraint and subtlety.[3] What was, I wondered, the purpose of such restraint? Could we think of it as Appelfeld's personal, stylistic signature? Or was this, perhaps, not just a matter of literary style but rather a rhetorical-behavioral pattern testifying, in a poetic way, to the presence of a deep traumatic core? What mechanism is responsible for producing textual restraint, and what purpose does it serve? And what are the poetic devices deployed to produce this effect?

During my work on Appelfeld's text, I realized that the more apparent the restraint in the text, the more charged the materials at hand, seeking to break out. I then proposed that this might be a way of regulating powerful underlying emotion: a poetic representation reflecting a textual struggle between two opposing forces: the destructive forces that might cause a collapse of textual coherence and the force for preservation of the text.

DOI: 10.4324/9781003403753-10

Poetic language is commonly considered to break the conventions of language and patterns of reality, moving into the unknown territory authors seek to reveal. The literary encounter with the unique phenomenon of the Holocaust, however, involves the extreme and radical. I therefore sought to approach poetic language from the opposite direction: from the perspective not of its fragmenting and subverting potential, but rather in so far as it enables to contain the catastrophic experience in the text, even though here the line to the ghostly domain of trauma is crossed. I studied the restraining qualities without which the annihilating powers of trauma would have overwhelmed the text.

This was the stage in my research when I looked for the meaning of Appelfeld's stylistic restraint and the mechanism that produced it. I mentioned four types of textual manifestations: reduction, indistinctness/blurring of domains, splitting, and equivalency. I assumed that together, these textual phenomena produced a blunting or muting effect, which made it possible to integrate the terrible events by resisting or refusing to convey them. These are the elements responsible for the feeling of "lost in the fog," and the sense of suffocation and oppression I experienced as a reader.

I continued to expand my study of restraint, trying to find out whether other possible poetic strategies for representing trauma had been used by other writers who also addressed the Holocaust. With this in mind I next looked at the work of Ka-Tzetnik and then Primo Levi. It was obvious that these writers used very divergent strategies to approach the memory of the traumatic experience and bear poetic witness to it. Here was a range of coping strategies, ranging between physical, bodily traumatic memory, emotional traumatic memory, and rational traumatic memory. Each of them included various formal devices keeping the text safe against collapse, employing them to varying extents; in all of these it was possible to identify what I later called "poetic defense mechanisms."

Poetic defense mechanisms are a metaphoric construct: they are second-order in the sense that texts are not living organisms. As a product, and extension, of the writing psyche, the poetic text creates a virtual space sufficiently detached from experience itself; as such, it makes psychic processing possible. These poetic defense mechanisms do not entertain one-to-one relations with psychic mechanisms. Bringing about transformation, the poetic text, by observing aesthetic distance from experience and due to the poetic devices the author uses in the emergent space, can touch upon the very heart of the matter, reaching zones which may well have remained out of reach otherwise.

A poetic text seeks to extend beyond what has been broken, to touch the traumatic core, the concrete essence of being – but it equally aims to represent that essence in the symbolic domain. This is achieved by means of processing, transformation, and reconstructing a new reality. The poetic text, in this sense, has a dual-code process and takes two complementary directions: while aiming to make contact with experience, it also observes and represents it. Though the drive for concreteness in relation to trauma is not without its risks and dangers, it is distinctly where a sense of authenticity may emerge. This is the scream that seeks its way out to be heard from behind the bars of reason, the urge to give voice to powerful emotion. It threatens to "burst" the text, and through a pendulum movement, an entire range of poetic devices is brought into play, which holds out a form that may contain the scream without the text collapsing into chaos.

This is to say that restraint is not a mere matter of style: it is the mechanism that creates the form so that the out-cry may occur, the site where the explosive forces of the scream meet with the text's poetic devices, the site at which it is possible to raise the worst of all without collapsing into chaos.

So, I replaced the search for Appelfeld's restraint as a merely aesthetic-rhetorical choice – and began thinking of it as a type of poetic textual defense mechanism embedded in each personal preference. This is what enabled the writers to put into words unspeakable experiences while keeping the text intact. The same goes for the novel by Ka-Tzetnik to which I then turned my attention, as well as to Primo Levi's work.

Form for a Scream

"Even then we understood screaming would not suffice. A form must be found, or else the scream would sound like madness, or worse: fake," wrote Appelfeld.[4] This book's central question is, indeed, what form the outcry should take in order for a text dealing with traumatic experience to steer clear of sounding either mad or worse: inauthentic. In my analyses, I have shown that coping with the trauma can be considered from two perspectives: one involves content and psychology and relates to the processing of trauma. The other concerns the formal and aesthetic, and it includes the modes of representation of these coping mechanisms in the rhetorical-poetic sense.

In her *Bearing Witness to the Witness*, Dana Amir presents a psychoanalytic investigation of different ways in which trauma is conveyed. She identifies four basic modes: metaphoric, metonymic, psychotic-excessive, and Muselmann-psychotic. What distinguishes these four modes is the respective distance between the experiencing self and the one who bears witness. It is, she argues, this distance that determines the extent to which the experience is processed in the act of bearing witness.[5]

In this book, I have studied different styles of mental coping with traumatic experience by looking at poetic representations. My approach to poetic texts of witnessing is aesthetic and psychoanalytic. Aesthetic, because rather than with conceptual materials, my main concern lies with the form, patterns, and modes of expression of these materials. I study the intricacies of the psyche as they are rendered in language through an analysis of poetic language: imagery, symbols, narratives, structures, and descriptive textures the writers, as artists, used when coping with trauma. This is why I pay close attention to style, rhetoric, symbolization, the use or avoidance of causal-logical implicature, and it is the reason why I discuss styles of writing such as restraint, kitsch, or rational-scientific forms. But this study of poetic form is nevertheless closely tied to the issue of psychic coping and of the traumatic reality. Poetic writing, which includes all the above-discussed strategies and patterns, can protect the psyche from trauma's destructive effect. And so, the aesthetic-poetic discussion throughout this book is two-pronged: It offers a consideration of the various modes of coping shown by a person who experienced trauma, as well as a discussion of the modes of textual coping presented by someone who writes about traumatic experience in a poetic way.

Psychological Discussion: Types of Coping with Trauma

My textual analysis yielded three styles of mental coping with the memory of a traumatic Holocaust experience: coping through body memory, coping through emotional memory, and coping by means of a rational memory. Body memory involves a type of coping where traumatic memory is stored on a primary level. As we saw in Chapter 2, Appelfeld preserved the traumatic memory in this dimension: "Everything that happened is imprinted within my body and not within my memory."[6]

In Appelfeld's case, terror was imprinted on the cellular level and became part of his body, like his arms or legs. I showed how poetic devices – reduction, blunting, dissociation, and equivalency – keep the information in the text on a low level of organization, situating it at a pre-categorical stage, which allows an approach to, and suggests contact with, the traumatic core by means of body memories.

While Appelfeld remains in the realm of the invisible subject and avoids conceptualizing the body experience, Ka-Tzetnik, by contrast, channels his experience via characters doomed to destruction through madness and suicide; he portrays this in terms of an explosive emotionality. Giving free rein to his experience of terror, this is what directed and imposed his particular mode of coping. His style is amplification: emotion is accentuated, and there is no way of controlling it. Here the emotions overrule everything else to the point of explosion.

It was Primo Levi's choice to cope with trauma by preserving it as a memory, reported and documented in a rational and controlled manner. He felt a powerful need to restore order, impose it on chaos, and explain – to both himself and others – why things were as they were. His rationalism enabled him to stay in control of the trauma he had suffered: "Writing is a way of creating order"[7] he said. Levi tried in his own way to find release from trauma – a journey which eventually defeated him.

What these texts preserving the memory of trauma have in common, over and beyond their different psychic strategies, is a notable lack of integration among the various systems: body, feeling, and consciousness. In some, trauma resulted in dissociation and blockage; in others it led to intensification and amplification. This destabilized the balance between systems. Each writer, in his own specific way, ended up in a situation where one system blocked or overwhelmed the others. The various patterns of mental coping with trauma discussed, showed how trauma ordained the subject to seek for release, a search which left him time and again, relentlessly and irredeemably, ensnared by it and by his personal mode of coping. The works studied, without exception, manifested the vulnerability and sense of shock typical of trauma.

The three authors struggled valiantly with the intense emotion trauma unleashes upon the self. While Appelfeld approaches feelings and touches them, almost reaching a level of conceptualization, then, however, to refuse to name and recognize; Levi deals with feelings by rationally restraining them, declining to look at them directly through most of his writing, while Ka-Tzetnik, by contrast, gives free rein to emotions to the point that his text nearly collapses under the burden.

Psychological analysis yields some insight into how the mind deploys its various defense mechanisms. It addresses the following question: What is the protective shield these authors chose in their respective encounters with trauma as they were writing these texts? What is their typical rhetoric? Did they, in the act of bearing witness, describe experience as an eternal, forever unresolvable present, or did they tell the story from the perspective of one who has processed the experience and transformed it into something of the past, from which one can then find release? Was experience conveyed by acting out or by working-through?

At the outset of my study, I assumed that Ka-Tzetnik's outcry, ostensibly unrestrained, represented a form of acting out, while Appelfeld's and Levi's obviously restrained texts represented types of working-through. I believed mechanisms of restraint reflected processing, testifying to engagement with poetic representation of the remembered experience of trauma. But analysis revealed a different, more complex picture. Ka-Tzetnik's novel *House of Dolls* did indeed display textual acting out and gave vent to an endless scream. Ka-Tzetnik's scream conveyed hysterical and obsessive amplification, was excessively verbose, and was burdened with an overload of imagery in its attempt to bring the traumatic past back into the present and stir powerful responses in his readers. Appelfeld's and Levi's respective styles, by comparison, are sober, leading me to conclude they were the result of working-through. But on closer inspection, this apparent working-through appeared more closely akin to acting out. In both Levi's and Appelfeld's cases acting out took the shape of negation, or refusal. There was, on the one hand, the refusal to conceptualize and give a name to the experience, as we saw in the case of Appelfeld's writing, and on the other, the refusal to deal with the unconscious and irrational aspects of existence, in Levi's case. Appelfeld's refusal to conceptualize led to a dissociation between the emotional and cognitive, a rejection of any generalization. Appelfeld chose to remain tethered to the body's experience, which was then resurrected time and again by means of emotion. Levi, unlike him, tended to split between reason and emotion. We may therefore argue that for each of these authors the traumatic experience made some kind of mental release impossible – each in their own manner: whether by excess and amplification, or by refusal and silencing: each remained trapped in his trauma.[8]

Literary Discussion: Poetic Defense Mechanisms

While the psychological part of my study looked at the relations between text and psychological defense mechanisms at work when coping with trauma, the literary discussion related to various formal or stylistic manifestations, i.e., restraint, kitsch, and scientific literacy, in the representation of traumatic memories. As said, the poetic text constitutes a safe place that keeps trauma at a safe distance, creating a system of checks and balances by means of which the harrowing experience can be mentioned while averting the risk of being totally consumed. The poetic testimony is equipped with a mechanism that controls distance from actual experience, something which creates what we know as "aesthetic distance."[9] Much like in rituals or in psychotherapy, a text can present the most terrifying experiences from a safe vantage point. The myth of Perseus and Medusa illustrates this: Anyone who looked directly at Medusa was doomed to die, but if her image was faced in the mirroring shield this fate would be averted. If there was any processing in these texts, it was through the poetic language whose textual defense mechanisms made it possible to render the horror and contain it.

Even though the different modes of coping of the authors whose work I discussed did not lead to some psychological redemption or release from the trauma, poetic language enabled them to contain, recount, and write the experience. All three produced a poetic envelope that served as a defense mechanism in the encounter with the experience. In Appelfeld's case this was restraint, which worked like a barrier between emotion and conceptualization, while for Levi it was scientific restraint that put a barrier between reason and feeling. But even Ka-Tzetnik needed something to block the destructive powers active in his work. I showed how he used, even if unconsciously, kitsch's ornamental aspect and its banal metaphoricity. While this resulted in emotional amplification, it also afforded poetic containment. Kitsch, by covering and enveloping trauma, saved the text from madness, but at the price of authenticity.

Traumatic Memory in Poetic Language

The Holocaust exceeds the parameters of ordinary reality. In the absence of any category that could serve to examine it, it is outside the domain of our senses, the imagination, or reason. All three of the authors studied here present trauma as a negative sublime, producing a psychological position of deep distress and uncontainable terror. Holocaust survivors, in this sense, endure an ongoing event which has no closure. As a result, it invades everything and is present everywhere.[10] How is such a remembered-unremembered memory to be represented by means of poetic language?

Poetic language operates at the boundaries, in the liminal regions of language. From this position it challenges language's occluding mechanisms. As I have been showing throughout this book, and following Kristeva, poetic language has a dual-code quality: It may question the fixed symbolic order by creating a crack through which shows the real: the domain of lack, of trauma. It can accomplish this without having to pay the price of crossing into the dangerous territory of madness or falsehood. But it also has the potential of rebuilding, reconstituting the broken domain of lack, and producing new, structured meaning within the symbolic order. Kristeva defines the praxis of poetic language as both acknowledgment of the law of the symbolic and its infringement for the purpose of renewal.[11] It is poetic language that is responsible for the dynamic movement between acting-out and working-through; this is a dynamic that results in a higher degree of freedom, releasing the writing self from entrapment in the fixation of trauma.

Poetic Language in Appelfeld, Levi, and Ka-Tzetnik

As the authors I have been discussing differed individually in terms of their coping with trauma, their ways of operating textual defense mechanisms in the service of poetic writing, too, diverged. While the brunt of Levi's restraint mechanism was invested in the structuring of trauma with a view to the symbolic order, Appelfeld put most of his effort into the fragmenting power of poetic expression, making sure all the while to stay within the boundaries of language.

For Levi it was "scientific" or objective restraint that allowed him to examine and assess reality in a controlled and rational manner. The aesthetic detachment afforded by scientific, mythic, and conceptual metaphors also helped to generate a literary defense zone. Restraint provided him with a sense of order and control in a chaotic reality.

Appelfeld went to the farthest, still articulate reaches of emotional restraint in order to touch upon the traumatic core. Restraint served to help in the reductive action to first strip language of its symbols and then to resurrect it by paying heed to its concrete properties: sound, voice, rhythm, and melody. He chose to preserve trauma in close proximity to the real. This choice for body memory seeks to hold on to something of the uncontrollability and the unconscious nature of terror and despair. While taking things to the very cusp of conceptualization,[12] Appelfeld eventually remains with condensed but unspoken emotion, unfocused feeling which defies categorization. He replaced focused, rational concepts with a language marked by an uncategorical indistinctness, dominated by tone, music, and rhythm, which is what produces the sense of being "lost in the fog." In this sense not only memory's content is of the body, but also its representation in language: Appelfeld's language is semiotic. It constitutes the traces of trauma. It unsettles the symbolic order and aims to represent trauma at the level of expression at its most reduced, barring silence. For him, it is only poetic language with its mechanisms of restraint that can touch the "molecules of suffering," and that can redeem trauma from the dimension of darkness. In his own words:

> Who will redeem from the darkness the fears, the pains, and the agony, the hidden beliefs, the sense of nothingness and the sense of eternity. Who will bring them out of the darkness and give them a little warmth and dignity, if not art.[13]

In the foregoing chapters I have argued that the mechanism of restraint acts against the destructive forces of trauma, producing the kind of homeostasis that transforms the traumatic experience into language. These forces – trauma's forces of fragmentation and rupture and the forces of preservation by contrast – are not on individual display in these texts. What we observe is their relative proportion, determined in each case by how the drive to fragmentation stands to the drive to preserve. Restraint can take many forms of modification inherent to poetic language itself. This is how the reader is exposed to the writer's traumatic experience as a function of the latter's poetic choices.

In the context of both Appelfeld's and Levi's restraint, Ka-Tzetnik's kitsch presents itself as somewhat of a riddle. Can we consider kitsch, with its characteristic excess, as a type of restraint, nevertheless? How can such stylistic behavior be considered a textual defense strategy? How can we look at Ka-Tzetnik's text as an illustration of how, even at its most tempestuous and extreme, poetic language preserves experience and passes it on to other witnesses. When, in court, it had to manage without its poetic defense mechanisms, Ka-Tzetnik's text indeed collapsed. But in the domain of poetic language, Ka-Tzetnik's text does not collapse. Here he uses textual defense mechanisms, with kitsch the foremost of his devices. This would seem a strange stylistic choice. He represents the traumatic experience by means of a style which has been called an "aesthetics of deception" – a style that deeply clashes with the shattered and boundless character of trauma. Ka-Tzetnik did not shy away from contact with trauma and looked at it open-eyed. But the stronger the outcry, the more strength he needed to keep it in control. His "choice of control" in representing the phenomenon, the use of kitsch as a style, exposes how he situated himself between the two forces: the wish to shatter and to destroy, and the wish to preserve. Ka-Tzetnik's text adheres to the style of kitsch, offering no escape or mode of processing, yet it is still "wrapped" by a defense mechanism of its own. It might be an unconscious choice, but one that shows a need for a kind of restraint, wrapping the abyss in aesthetic covers like "beautiful death."

Maurice Blanchot describes the creative act in reference to the story of Orpheus' descent into the underworld, determined to set free Eurydice. He discusses the profound experience of the underworld while insisting on avoiding exaggeration by being restrained, controlled, and indirect: "The deep does not reveal itself directly [...]."[14]

And so, we come back to the myth of Perseus, who, in order to look at the horror of the Medusa, used his mirroring shield with its double code: protection against the horror as well as the possibility of coping with it. Similarly, the authors discussed in this book, whose real-life conditions forced them to use a psychic strategy that prevented a type of working-through, were able to manage, in their poetic world, using their respective, unique poetic style, to tell and pass on the story of their trauma by way of poetic testimony. Combining shield and mirror, using poetic language, each was able to produce a finely spun fabric that contained the horrible experience. And so, it was represented in spite of everything and was successfully communicated to others, rather than collapsing into chaos.

Notes

1 Aharon Appelfeld, "Beyond Tragedy", *First Person Essays* (World Zionist Organization, 1979), 49. [Hebrew].
2 W. G. Sebald, KCRW Interview Bookworm. W. G. Sebald (6 December, 2001).
3 See my Appelfeld chapter.

4 Appelfeld, "Beyond Tragedy", 49. [Hebrew; translated by Mirjam Meerschwam Hadar].
5 Dana Amir, *Bearing Witness to the Witness* (Routledge, 2019).
6 Aharon Appelfeld, *The Story of a Life* (Knopf Doubleday Publishing Group., Kindle Edition), 89.
7 Roberto Di Caro, "The Essential and the Superfluous in the Voice of Memory", in *Primo Levi, Interviews 1961–1987* (The New York Press, 2001), 174.
8 Rina Dudai, *Modes of Coping with Trauma in Holocaust Literature (A. Appelfeld, Ka-Tzetnik, P. Levi)* (doctoral dissertation, Hebrew University of Jerusalem, 2000). [Hebrew]; a similar discussion also appears in Yochai Atira, "Death of the Witness in the Age of Witnessing", *Ma'arag 6* (2006) The Magness Press, 177–214. [Hebrew].
9 Edward Bullough, "Psychical Distance as a Factor in Art and an Aesthetic Principle", *British Journal of Psychology 5:2* (1912), 87–118.
10 Dori Laub, "Bearing Witness, or the Vicissitudes of Listening," in *Testimony, Crises of Witnessing in Literature, Psychoanalysis, and History*, eds. Shoshana Felman and Dori Laub (Routledge, 1992), 69.
11 Julia Kristeva, *Revolution in Poetic Language*, trans. Margaret Waller (Columbia University Press, 1984), 194–235.
12 Kristeva, *Revolution in Poetic Language.*
13 Aharon Appelfeld, *First Person Essays* (World Zionist Organization, 1979), 98. [Hebrew; English translation by Mirjam Meerschwam Hadar].
14 Maurice Blanchot, "The Gaze of Orpheus", in *The Space of Literature*, trans. Ann Smock (University of Nebraska Press, 1989), 171–176.

References

Amir, Dana, *Bearing Witness to the Witness* (Routledge, 2019).

Appelfeld, Aharon, "Beyond Tragedy", in *First Person Essays* (World Zionist Organization, 1979), 49. [Hebrew].

Appelfeld, Aharon, *The Story of a Life* (Knopf Doubleday Publishing Group., Kindle Edition, 2004), 89–90.

Atira, Yochai, "Death of the Witness in the Age of Witnessing", *Ma'arag 6* (2006) The Magness Press, 177–214. [Hebrew].

Blanchot, Maurice, *The Space of Literature*, trans. Ann Smock (University of Nebraska Press, [1955] 1989), 171–176.

Bullough, Edward, "Psychical Distance as a Factor in Art and an Aesthetic Principle", *British Journal of Psychology 5:2* (1912), 87–118.

Celan, Paul, "Speech on the Occasion of Receiving the Literature Prize of the Free Hanseatic City of Bremen", in *Selected Poems and Prose of Paul Celan*, trans. John Felstiner (W.W. Norton, [1958] 2001), 395–396.

Di Caro, Roberto, "The Essential and the Superfluous in the Voice of Memory", in Belpoliti Marco and Gordon Robert, eds., *Primo Levi, Interviews 1961–1987* (The New York Press, 2001), 167–175.

Dudai, Rina, *Modes of Coping with Trauma in Holocaust Literature (A. Appelfeld, Ka-Tzetnik, P. Levi)* (doctoral dissertation, Hebrew University of Jerusalem, 2000). [Hebrew].

Kristeva, Julia, *Revolution in Poetic Language*, trans. Margaret Waller (Columbia University Press, 1984), 194–235.

Laub, Dori, "Bearing Witness, or the Vicissitudes of Listening," in Shoshana Felman and Dori Laub, eds., *Testimony, Crises of Witnessing in Literature, Psychoanalysis, and History* (Routledge, 1992), 69.

Sebald, W. G., Interview with Michael Silverblatt, Bookworm, KCRW (Santa Monica. Radio broadcast, 6 December, 2001).

Index

Note: Page numbers followed by 'n' refer to notes.

For Product Safety Concerns and Information please contact our EU representative GPSR@taylorandfrancis.com Taylor & Francis Verlag GmbH, Kaufingerstraße 24, 80331 München, Germany